Animal Bones

ANIMAL BONES

James Rackham

Published for the Trustees of the British Museum
by British Museum Press

Acknowledgements

I would like to thank my wife for reading a draft of the text and for her many helpful comments, and John Casey for initially introducing me to the idea of this small volume. I am grateful to Don Brothwell and Sheridan Bowman for comments and corrections and to Nina Shandloff for her helpful guidance from start to finish. The following kindly supplied photographs: Arthur MacGregor (**3**); Museum of London (**2, 5, 11, 12, 40**); Henry Bunn (**19**); George Frison (**25**); Bodil Bratlund, Archäologisches Landesmuseum, Schleswig (**26**); British Museum, Ian Riddler, Robert White (**37, 39**); Colleen Batey (**38**).

Figure references

Cover illustration after M. Maitland Howard, The Skeleton Hunt, in I. W. Cornwall, *Bones for the Archaeologist* (1974), p. 12 (courtesy J. M. Dent & Sons Ltd); **13** after J.-M. Cordy, Palaeoecology of the Late Glacial and early Postglacial of Belgium and neighbouring areas, *The Late Glacial in north-west Europe* (1991), fig. 5.4, p. 45; **16** after A. Stuart, *Pleistocene Vertebrates in the British Isles* (1982), fig. 9.1, pp. 168–9; **17** after B. Gordon, *Of Men and Reindeer herds in French Magdalenian Prehistory* (1989), fig. 27, p. 87; **18** after G. Isaac, The diet of early man, *World Archaeology 2* (1971), pp. 278–98; **19** from H. T. Bunn, Evidence on the diet and subsistence patterns of plio-pleistocene hominids at Koobi Fora, Kenya, and Olduvai Gorge, Tanzania, *Animals and Archaeology 1* (1983), fig. 1(B), p. 24; **20** data from L. Binford, *Faunal Remains from Klasies River Mouth* (1984), table 3.6, p. 89; **21** after M. Street, Bedburg-Königshoven: a Pre-boreal Mesolithic site in the Lower Rhineland, Germany, *The Late Glacial in north-west Europe* (1991), fig. 24.6, p. 264; **22, 23** after A. Legge and P. Rowley-Conwy, *Star Carr Revisited* (1988), fig. 7, p. 23 and fig. 37, p. 83; **24** data from J. Speth, *Bison kills and Bone counts* (1983), table 11, p. 75; **26** from B. Bratlund, A study of hunting lesions containing flint fragments on reindeer bones at Stellmoor, Schleswig-Holstein, Germany, *The Late Glacial in north-west Europe* (1991), fig. 18.2, p. 195; **27** after F. Audouze and J. Enloe, Subsistence strategies and economy in the Magdalenian of the Paris Basin, France, *The Late Glacial in north-west Europe* (1991), fig. 8.1, p. 66; **28** after R. Meadow, Animal Domestication in the Middle East: A view from the Eastern margin, *Animals and Archaeology 3* (1984), fig. 1, p. 317; **29** data from J. Wheeler, On the origin and early development of Camelid pastoralism in the Andes, *Animals and Archaeology 3* (1984), table 1, p. 398; **30** after B. Hesse, These are our goats: the origins of herding in West Central Iran, *Animals and Archaeology 3* (1984), fig. 1, p. 252; **31** after C. Grigson, Size and sex – evidence for the domestication of cattle in the Near East, *The Beginnings of Agriculture* (1989), fig. 5, p. 93; **32** data from J. Bourdillon and J. Coy, The animal bones, *Excavations at Melbourne Street, Southampton 1971–76* (1978), table 17.1, p. 81; **34** data from T. O'Connor, Bones from 46–54 Fishergate, *The Archaeology of York, The Animal Bones 15/4*, table 74, p. 265.

Designed by Andrew Shoolbred

Set in Compugraphic Palacio and printed in
Great Britain by The Bath Press, Avon

ISBN 0-7141-2057-X

A catalogue record for this book is available from
the British Library

Cover illustration A bone analyst's perspective on a hunter and his horse, taken from a fanciful tableau entitled 'The Skeleton Hunt'.

Contents

Preface

The bones of animals are one of the most common finds on many archaeological excavations and as such they have been studied by zoologists and archaeologists for many years. In addition to their intrinsic interest as evidence of the occurrence of animals, both domestic and wild, in various places and times throughout human history, they can also yield information that helps us to interpret our past just as artefacts such as pottery and metalwork do.

In a volume of this size one cannot hope to present all aspects of a field of study, and if readers wish to pursue the subject they could do worse than to start with the books mentioned under Further Reading (page 63). Nevertheless, I hope to convey the wide range of information that can be gathered through the study of animal bones and to draw attention to some of the problems. New developments occur quite regularly and lead to new techniques and interpretations, and one of the exciting aspects of the work is these fresh ideas.

I have chosen to illustrate the subject by presenting a series of examples which I believe are particularly good or convenient for explaining a method of analysis or interpretation. The work of the original researchers is noted by chapter on page 63, and a separate list of figure references is given for all the data illustrated. These examples, though drawn from a wide geographic area, are of necessity limited; many of the methods of analysis are as pertinent to one period of study as they are to another, so the same techniques are applied on most sites, although interpretations may differ.

I have used a number of terms that geologists and archaeologists employ to describe periods and cultures. These will probably be unfamiliar to many readers, but they are preferable to constant repetition of 10,000 years ago or 500,000 years ago, which would become tedious. Figure **15** (on page **28**) presents a chronology for all such terms and the sites mentioned in the text.

I hope in presenting this brief introduction to a large and diverse subject that readers will derive some enjoyment and even amazement from what can be discovered about long-dead animals and the human societies that hunted or kept them.

— 1 —

What Can a Bone Tell Us?

Interpreting the past through archaeological remains depends upon the identification and detailed analysis of evidence collected during excavation. This may take the form of records of the soil removed and subsequently discarded, or it may be the study of the items collected. Datable and durable artefacts such as pottery or coins can obviously contribute to the understanding of a site and thus to our knowledge of life in the past, but it may not be so immediately apparent what can be learned from the investigation of animal bones.

We will consider first the possible information contained within a single bone, or even a fragment of bone. Studied in turn, these individual bones or fragments are the building blocks of our knowledge of the past. While some may yield little or no information, others indirectly can tell us of time, climate, environment, farming, butchery, religion and trade. The information amassed from these small pieces of evidence can then be amalgamated and used to paint a much broader picture.

The identification of a bone

The animal skeleton is designed (or has evolved) to fulfil a function which combines protection, support and locomotion. While the animal kingdom is made up of many diverse groups, there is a surprisingly uniform skeletal pattern within each of the five groups or classes of bony animals (vertebrates): fishes, amphibians, reptiles, birds and mammals. The five classes vary in their skeleton in a manner particular to their evolution and lifestyle and it is this consistency within each class that allows a particular bone fragment to be identified to the correct skeletal element, whatever the individual species. Nevertheless, not all the excavated fragments retain sufficient of the characteristic parts of a whole bone to make correct identification possible.

Identifications are made on the basis of the morphology (shape) of each bone (fig. 1), as its structure varies in relation to its function in the body. Long bones – the cylindrical bones forming the main elements of the limbs – are mainly comprised of a hollow tube of solid bone to which is attached at each end a separately growing piece of bone, an epiphysis, which carries an articulation (bearing sur-

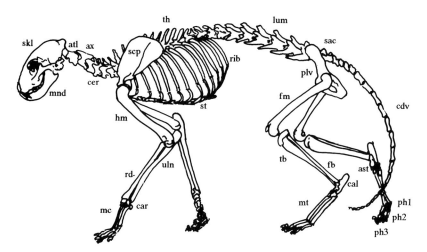

1 The main bones of the mammal skeleton (using a cat as the model). The mammalian skeleton has about 200 bones and comprises the skull, vertebrae and ribs, and the bones of the limbs. Except when whole skeletons are found, the individual bones rarely occur intact, generally breaking into a number of pieces. The following bones are labelled: **skl** (skull), **mnd** (mandible), **atl** (atlas), **ax** (axis), **cer** (cervical vertebrae), **th** (thoracic vertebrae), **lum** (lumbar vertebrae), **sac** (sacrum), **cdv** (caudal vertebrae), **scp** (scapula), **hm** (humerus), **rd** (radius), **uln** (ulna), **car** (carpals), **mc** (metacarpus), **ph1** (phalanx 1), **ph2** (phalanx 2), **ph3** (phalanx 3), **rib** (rib), **st** (sternum), **plv** (pelvis), **fm** (femur), **tb** (tibia), **fb** (fibula), **cal** (calcaneum), **ast** (astragalus), **mt** (metatarsus).

face) with which the end (articulation) of the next bone normally forms a rotating joint. These articulations may be in the form, very simply, of a ball-and-socket joint (as in the shoulder and hip joints), which can rotate in three dimensions, or grooved articulations (as in the knee and elbow), which only move in two dimensions. These functional needs determine the shape of the joint and hence help us to identify from which joint a fragment derives. Other bones such as those of the wrist, ankle and spine take compressive forces while the animal is moving and are therefore blockish, normally with a network of spongy bone within, rather than hollow. Yet other bones – such as the ribs, shoulder blades, pelvic bones and skull – tend to be broad, flat bones designed to protect the soft organs within the body from damage.

While all these basic anatomical characteristics can help in recognising which bone a fragment comes from, the final test is to compare the pieces with real examples. Any skeleton from a modern animal of similar size to the archaeological specimen is adequate to assist in or confirm the identification. With time and persistence even very small fragments, with no obvious diagnostic character, may be identified, but this is rarely worth the effort because the next stage – identification of the species – may never be possible.

So, having established which bone of the body it is, the next step is to identify from which species it comes (fig. **2**). Size is one of the most important factors, and most animals can be divided readily into size categories, i.e. birds the size of sparrows, pigeons, chickens, domestic geese, turkey or eagles; or mammals the size of mice, rabbits, sheep, cattle or rhinoceroses. Secondly, as mentioned above, their function in terms of evolution and lifestyle affects the morphology of bones. The artiodactyls (even-toed ungulates) – cattle, sheep and deer – are generally long-legged and walk on their toes, are very similar in appearance and

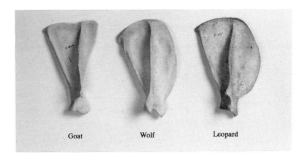

2 The scapulae (shoulder blades) of three species of mammal. These show the general uniformity of a bone element and yet illustrate the differences that allow the identification of each species. When a bone is fragmented it is necessary to record which parts are present and whether they are from the left or right side. In this way the minimum number of animals (MNI) in a sample can be estimated.

Goat   Wolf   Leopard

have a reduced number of digits in their feet. In contrast, mammals of the order Carnivora, such as dogs, bears and cats, move differently – walking on the pads of their feet – and normally have all five digits. Cattle are grazers, so their teeth reflect this habit, while carnivores, being flesh-eaters, need pointed or edged teeth for cutting the meat of their prey. Recognising these traits reduces the range of possibilities and often the fragment will only need to be compared with two or three reference species. Common sense obviously also plays a part; for instance, the fragment is always matched first against animals whose range is known to include the area of the site before it is compared with more exotic species. Even the most seemingly unpromising fragments can yield information on their bone and species origin to an experienced zooarchaeologist.

Sex and age

Although the species and bone type constitute the primary information from a fossil or archaeological bone, this is by no means the limit of the potential information. The sex of the animal, how old it was when it died, what time of year it died, and whether it was ill or injured may all be determinable, and almost certainly if the whole or a substantial part of the skeleton survives.

In determining the sex of an animal, many of its bones are of no use at all; others may permit a conclusion which is statistically valid, and yet others allow a categoric identification. Examples of the latter are the presence or absence of antlers in deer species, in which the females never – except in the case of reindeer – carry antlers; the size and character of the horns in some species (fig. **3**);

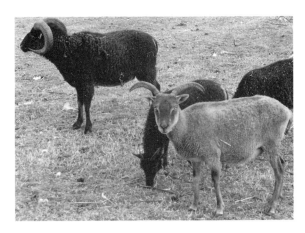

3 Adult male (*left*) and female Soay sheep, showing both the difference in the horn shape between the sexes and the typically larger size of the male.

9

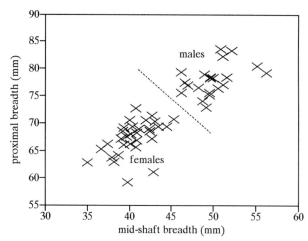

4 The scatterplot shows the distribution of two measurements taken on the metacarpus – a foot bone (see fig. **1**) – of the extinct bison, *Bison priscus*, collected from a gravel pit at Isleworth, west London. The bones are approximately 40,000 years old. Two clear groups can be differentiated on the plot and illustrate the size dimorphism between the sexes in the bison population at this period.

the presence, absence or size of tusks in animals such as pigs, hippopotamuses and walruses; and the presence or absence of spurs in some birds such as chickens and pheasants. A rather more subtle indicator of sex in many animals is the shape of the skull and pelvic bones.

While such anatomical features normally yield a secure identification, it is often rare for these bones to occur sufficiently intact in archaeological collections, so these methods may be of little use. However, many animal species show a difference in size between the sexes (fig. **3**), one sex being significantly larger than the other, which is exhibited by all or most of the bones of the skeleton. It is therefore possible from certain measurements on particular bones to illustrate this size difference and therefore identify the sex of the animals to which the individual bones belonged (fig. **4**). These data allow the assignment of bones to sex at an acceptable statistical level. More importantly for subsequent interpretation, the researcher is likely to have enough measurements to estimate the relative proportions of each sex in the archaeological sample.

It is generally possible to sex only the bones of adult animals, which raises the question of how we can recognise adults – or for that matter estimate the age – of any animals from their bones. This is possible because the skeleton is designed to increase in size during growth without prejudicing the functional needs of the animal. Bone is a living tissue and can increase in both length and girth.

The most useful fragments for establishing how old an animal was are the upper and lower jaws (maxilla and mandible). These carry the teeth, which in all mammals undergo a sequence of eruption, wear and loss. The process of replacement of the deciduous or baby teeth by an adult dentition can last for a number of years (fig. **5**). Subsequent wear on the teeth can also be used to establish the relative or approximate age of adult animals. If a whole jaw is found, the developmental age of the animal can often be estimated quite accurately. The classic phrase 'don't look a gift-horse in the mouth' refers to this ability to age an animal from the wear on its teeth – the inference being that if you are not asked to pay for the horse it is impolite to check its age.

Not only the teeth can be used. In a young mammal, the ends (epiphyses) of the long bones are attached to their shafts by cartilage. This becomes converted to bone over a period of time, fusion of the articulation to the shaft becoming complete when the bone ceases to grow in length. This ossification takes place in different joints at different ages (fig. **6**), from soon after birth to five years or older.

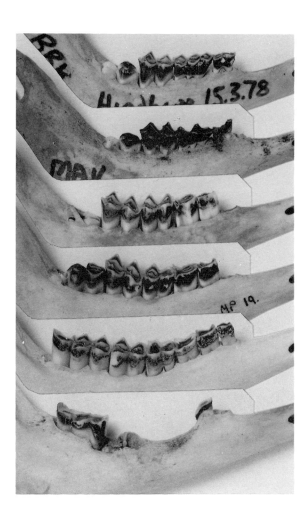

10 mths

1 yr

3 yrs

4 yrs

7 yrs

9 yrs

5 A collection of feral goat jaws from animals of different ages. The youngest jaws (*top*) have deciduous (baby) teeth, which are shed in the adult. The oldest animal (*bottom*) shows heavy wear on all its teeth and the loss of some molars. The complete adult dentition is often only in place after sexual maturity is reached; from this time on, age can only be assessed by the extent of wear on the different teeth.

6 (*below*) The fused (**F**) or unfused (**U**) condition of the epiphyses of a modern sample of feral goats from Scotland. The epiphyses are arranged in the approximate order in which they fused during life. As the animals become progressively older, a larger number of their epiphyses are fused. Hence an animal four years old will have all those epiphyses above the distal metatarsus fused, a number possibly fused or undergoing fusion and all those below the proximal ulnal epiphysis unfused. A goat metatarsus with the distal epiphysis unfused must come from an animal of less than four years, while a fragment with this part fused must derive from an individual aged three years or more. (See fig. 1 for the location of the bones; proximal (**p**) = end closest to spine; distal (**d**) = end furthest from spine.)

| | Age (in months) | | | | | | |
	12	24	36	48	60	72	108
distal humerus	F	F	F	F	F	F	F
proximal radius	F	F	F	F	F	F	F
scapula tuberosity	U/F	F	F	F	F	F	F
acetabular symphysis	U/F	F	F	F	F	F	F
proximal 2nd phalanx	U	U/F	F	F	F	F	F
proximal 1st phalanx	U	U/F	F	F	F	F	F
distal tibia	U	U	U/F	F	F	F	F
proximal femur	U	U	U/F	F	F	F	F
distal metacarpus	U	U	U/F	F	F	F	F
distal metatarsus	U	U	U/F	F	F	F	F
proximal calcaneum	U	U	U	U/F	F	F	F
distal femur	U	U	U	U/F	F	F	F
proximal tibia	U	U	U	U/F	F	F	F
distal radius	U	U	U	U/F	F	F	F
proximal humerus	U	U	U	U/F	U/F	F	F
proximal ulna	U	U	U	U/F	U/F	F	F
distal ulna	U	U	U	U	U/F	U/F	F
illial & ischial tub.	U	U	U	U	U/F	U/F	F
left & right pubis	U	U	U	U	U	U/F	F
vertebral centra	U	U	U	U	U	U/F	F

The sequence on the pelvis is a case in point. The pelvis is formed from six bones, three on either side of the body: the ilium, ischium and pubis. They fuse together at the articulation point (acetabular symphysis) with the femur very soon after birth because this is an important locomotory joint. The ilium and ischium carry tuberosities, roughened lumps of bone to which the muscles are attached. These fuse on to the body of the bones when the animals are young adults, and the final fusion of the left and right sides of the pelvic girdle may not happen until the animal is quite old.

If a complete skeleton is present, it is possible to establish precisely what developmental stage the animal had reached when it died. Where only single fragments occur with only one epiphysis, the age estimate is of the 'older than' or 'younger than' type. Nevertheless, the recording of this information allows the analyst to assign percentages of the archaeological sample to different age categories in a manner not dissimilar to modern census data (see fig. **35**). It is this amalgamation of data from a large sample of bones that is then interpreted, rather than the individual records.

The collection of a large set of data from the jaws of a species permits a similar, but more accurate, presentation of results than can be obtained from the epiphyseal data.

Individual animals in a population will reach a particular developmental stage, tooth eruption or epiphyseal fusion at slightly different ages due to natural variation, but the majority will reach it at broadly the same age.

Separate populations of the same species may sometimes differ by more significant amounts, particularly through genetic or nutritional variation. For instance, sheep in North America, Scotland or Turkey may develop at different rates, due to a variety of factors, and modern sheep, Roman sheep or Neolithic sheep may equally show this variability, particularly since selective breeding has taken place in many areas only over the last few hundred years. This means that while analysts traditionally give an age to individual archaeological examples, these are generally based upon ages obtained from modern European sheep flocks which, although accurate enough for analytical purposes, should therefore be considered approximate.

Season of death

Many of the behavioural and physiological activities of animals are seasonal in character. Mating, migration and birth generally take place during specific seasons, and the cycle of feeding and the availability of food are also seasonal in many parts of the world. The winter period is characteristically a time of little or no growth, while spring and early summer is normally a rapid growth period; autumn is the time when food resources are taken on in the form of fat deposits, so little growth takes place. Various aspects of the skeletons of all vertebrates reflect these behavioural and physiological changes.

Some of these are very easy to recognise. Female birds build up calcium deposits within the normally hollow long bones of their wings and legs just before laying, so that they can mobilise enough calcium to form the eggshell. By X-raying or drilling these bones to establish the presence or absence of these deposits, it is possible to ascertain whether female birds died during the laying season, generally a defined period for most species, or outside of this season. Similarly, deer develop their antlers during a short season before mating, carry

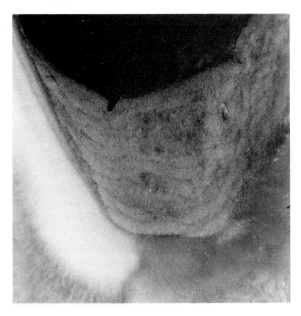

7 This photograph illustrates the cementum lines on the first molar of the jaw bone of a Roman ox from Castle Street, Carlisle. Cementum is laid down on the roots of the teeth. The pattern of growth is annual, with a light band showing the main period of growth and a thinner dark line indicating the winter. By counting the dark lines, the number of years the animal survived after the eruption of the tooth – at six to nine months of age – can be established. Nine dark bands can be seen, with perhaps a tenth forming on the extreme edge of the cementum. The animal therefore survived nine and a half years after the eruption of the first molar and was probably killed in the late autumn or early winter.

them during the rut, and shed them some weeks later. Therefore fragments of skull with or without antlers can indicate the part of this cycle – and therefore the time of year – in which the animal died (see fig. **22**).

Some of the bones and teeth of animals undergo a cycle of growth which leaves visible evidence within the tissue, in the form of lines that indicate a cessation of growth. The horns of temperate ruminants (cud-chewing mammals) are the clearest indication of this mechanism. Although rarely found in archaeological contexts, the pattern of growth illustrates the seasonal cycle. The major growth period, spring and summer, produces a marked growth in the size of the horn, but during autumn this diminishes, and it ceases in winter. This produces a sequence of bands, coincident with the winter, that enables both the age of the animal and the time of year within the cycle to be broadly established. The scales and otoliths (ear bones) of fishes and the teeth of mammals (fig. 7) are body parts which survive in archaeological deposits and within which this cycle of growth is sometimes visible. These can also be used to age the animals: the ox in figure **9**, for instance, was nearly eleven years old when it was slaughtered. These bands have not been recorded in all animals, but where visible either nutrition or physiological cycles are thought to control their formation. Such growth lines may be difficult to detect in domestic species maintained and fed year round.

The accuracy of these estimates of season is limited and is unlikely to be closer than within three months. While animals are still in their first year and their teeth are still erupting, it is normally possible to estimate the time of year they died by matching their teeth with those of modern animals whose age and season of death are known.

What else can we learn?

Much work has been carried out relating the measured size of bones to the size of the animal when alive, both in terms of height at the shoulder (or withers) and body weight. We have already seen that size can indicate sex, but peoples in the past may also have been interested in an animal's size for reasons of status or ritual, or simply for the amount of food on the carcass. Fish, particularly, vary in size considerably with age: a young cod might be 20 cm long and have a gutted weight of 0.07 kg, while the same fish could eventually reach a length of 100 cm and weigh 8.7 kg when gutted. The size of fish found on a site can therefore also give an indication of the fishing methods that might have been used, such as hooks or nets.

During life, animals may catch diseases, undergo periods of poor nutrition, be injured accidentally or in fights or even through hunting, and develop pathologies (changes to the bone) associated with genetic or environmental factors. This evidence, when present, can give some information on the life history of the animal. For example, if an animal is hobbled it may develop callouses on the lower limbs which produce changes to the bone. Some pathologies found on the feet of cattle are thought to result from the use of the animals as plough oxen or draught animals (fig. **8**). Bits on a horse harness may cause unusual wear on the teeth. Such factors may allow some comments on the function of animals during life. Healed injuries from hunting have been identified from prehistoric sites, including examples where a flint arrowhead has remained embedded in the bone and new bone has formed around it.

Perhaps the most exciting new technique for learning about a bone is that of DNA fingerprinting. Research has shown that DNA can be extracted from ancient material, such as bone. DNA sequences provide a genetic dictionary of an animal and hold the key to many of the relationships between individuals, populations and species. The successful development of DNA identification techniques will allow many new questions to be tackled. For example, we may be able to identify the origin of imported domestic animals – both the first prehistoric

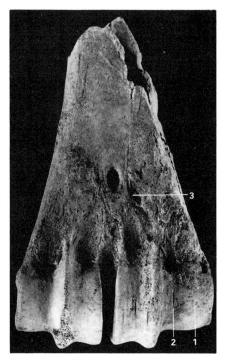

8 This medieval cattle metatarsus from Middlegate, Hartlepool, exhibits pathologies thought to be caused by the extra stresses experienced when animals are used as draught oxen. The articulation is expanded (**1**) and the joint surface is scored and grooved (**2**) by abrasion with the phalanges (toe bones). The inflammation thus caused in the joint has led to further bone formation (**3**).

14

introductions and later imports which accompanied succeeding migrations of people. We could establish whether particular species were domesticated in more than one area of the world. We might be able to study the antiquity and origin of breeds. We might even be able to discover the distances over which cattle and other stock were traded by identifying where they came from before they were driven to market in towns.

So far we have been concerned with the original animal and its life and characteristics, but we can also discover something of the person or people who killed, butchered or ate them. The bone may well carry physical evidence of butchery. Chop and cut marks are not infrequent on archaeological bones and it is possible to establish from microscopic study of the marks whether flint or metal tools or other mechanisms were responsible (see fig. **19**). Even greater refinement may be possible. Knife cuts, cleaver chops and saw marks are all readily recognisable from the form and character of the butchery marks. Some experts are even confident in identifying different types of flint tool marks. The location and angle of the butchery mark, in combination with the evidence for the type of tool, can inform us about the action that caused it. For instance, skinning characteristically leaves small, fine, surface cuts on the bones that lie immediately beneath the skin, like those of the feet or skull. Butchering of the carcass into units small enough to carry may produce cut marks on the surface of articulations where bones are attached by ligaments which were severed or broken to separate the bones. More extensive evidence of butchery may be present when bones have been chopped or cleaved into joint- or pot-sized cooking pieces, or where the shafts of long bones have been smashed to extract the marrow.

Evidence of butchery is not the only explanation for man-made marks on archaeological bones. Fresh animal bone has been a source of raw material for humans and early hominids for probably over a million years. Being harder than wood but more easily worked than stone, it has had many functional and decorative uses. Manufacturing marks may be visible on bone tools or decorative objects which allow identification of the craftsman's tool kit, although most of the fragments found on an excavation are in fact the waste from this working rather than the objects themselves (see fig. **39**).

We may be able to take the human history of a bone fragment even further. Evidence of cooking is mostly intangible from archaeological bone, but occasionally bone fragments occur in which just one end of the bone is blackened. It is possible that in many cases this reflects the slight charring of the bone protruding from a joint being roasted over a fire. Cooking of any sort, particularly boiling bones for gruel, breaks down the proteins and fats in the bone and leaches out the minerals. This loss of organic and mineral matter from the bone tissue changes its character, making it more porous and fragile, and hence reducing its chances of survival in the soil.

Finally, the bones may hold clues to their own history – that of the individual fragments. An animal may be butchered and its bones dispersed, chopped, boiled, burnt, thrown away, chewed by dogs and eroded by soil acids, weathering and other soil processes until they finally survive in a stable condition within an archaeological deposit. This history may be long and convoluted for a small, unidentifiable fragment of bone on an archaeological site with thousands of years of history.

Clearly, unravelling this history is a lot more complicated than, for instance, identifying the animal species, and single fragments can rarely tell a comprehensible part of this story. The condition, colour, texture, staining, weight and robustness of the fragment can be recorded and may in part reflect this history. Different parts of a bone survive better than others, so it is important to know exactly which part is present. If the bone has been in a fire, its colour, texture and weight change. Chemical studies can be carried out to measure the amount of surviving protein. All these variables are affected to some degree by what happened to the bone during its disposal and subsequent burial.

This is a surprisingly important aspect of the analysis of animal bones. Fundamentally, we are interested in establishing information from which we can interpret the life and environment of past societies. We must therefore be aware that the assemblages we study may have become seriously biased through the processes of decay, degradation and disturbance, and during the incorporation of the material into the archaeological deposits. To illustrate this at its simplest level, if bones are scavenged by dogs they are likely to eat most of the juvenile bones, which are softer than adult bones, while destroying a much smaller proportion of the harder adult bones. As a result, a high proportion of adults in an excavated sample would not in this instance be a true reflection of the contemporary evidence, but rather would be due to heavy bias caused by scavenging.

One example is presented here to illustrate some of what has been discussed above. Figure 9 is a bone which is readily identifiable as a jaw from the presence of teeth. Comparison with reference material confirms that it is an ox bone. All the teeth are adult and fairly well worn, indicating an old animal. Ten 'annual' lines visible in the cementum of the first molar indicate an age of about eleven years. The outer cementum band is wide and pale, suggesting that the animal was slaughtered during the growing season, probably in the summer. Unfortunately there are no characteristics that allow us to recognise what sex the animal was, although we know from experience that within any domestic husbandry regime it is unlikely that either bulls or bullocks would have been allowed to live to this age. That part of the jaw which articulates with the skull has been chopped, indicating removal of this bone from the skull by butchery, possibly associated with the extraction of the tongue. There are also heavy chop marks below the teeth. Lastly, the condition of the bone is very good: there has been no leaching or erosion and the bone was buried in deposits with well-preserved organic remains. This indicates little likelihood of disturbance after discard, and that the bone was probably close to or in its initial disposal location.

While the individual bone fragments and the information they yield are building blocks in the study of archaeological animal bones, most of our understanding of the past derives from the amalgamation of these data. This might include all the fragments from within a rubbish pit or from a single layer thought to have formed during a short or definable period of time, or it may include all the fragments from an entire archaeological site. The data collected from the individual bones are analysed in a variety of ways to assist the archaeologist's interpretations and these are discussed in later chapters.

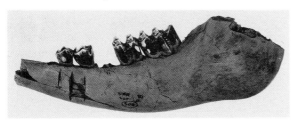

9 A cattle jaw recovered from excavations of Roman date just outside the Roman fort at Castle Street, Carlisle, England. The absent first molar was sectioned to study the cementum on the roots.

— 2 —

Bones and the Archaeologist

The serious study of fossil and archaeological bones began in the first half of the nineteenth century, although reports of fossil finds are recorded as early as 1676 with a reference to a thigh bone that was believed to belong to a female giant. One of the earliest accounts was of investigations at Kirkdale Cave, Yorkshire, by Dean William Buckland. His account was published in the *Philosophical Transactions of the Royal Society* in 1822 and was the prelude to a century of cave digging by Victorian vicars, scholars and amateurs alike. At this time the orthodox biblical view of the Creation was still widely accepted, and the finds of bones of extinct animals were assumed to predate the Flood. The following year, in 1823, Buckland published a book entitled *Reliquiae Diluvianae* ('Relics of the Flood') in which he wrote up his excavations of a number of caves (fig. **10**).

The traditional view was held with such fervour that any association of flint tools with these extinct animals was denied, even when they were found together in subsequent cave excavations. The tools were believed to be intrusions, or to have been mixed with the bones through the action of the Flood. It was not until after the middle of the century, when the combined efforts of Darwin, Huxley and others had changed the philosophical climate sufficiently for the antiquity of humankind to be accepted, that William Pengelly and Hugh Falconer published an account of work at Brixham Cave, England, where they found flint artefacts associated with the bones of woolly mammoths and other beasts. Bones became a major area of academic research and a number of well-illustrated accounts of finds from caves and gravel and brick pits were published.

In the latter half of the century this interest was tapped by archaeologists such as General Pitt-Rivers, whose excavation accounts include reports on the identification of the animal bones he found. The reporting of bones from archaeological sites continued into the twentieth century, and a great many accounts were published from sites all over Europe. These reports were generally of a descriptive rather than an interpretive nature, written by zoologists and palaeontologists at a time when the classification of species (taxonomy) and comparative anatomy were the favoured topics of the day.

Reports of this sort continued to be published right up to the 1950s, when the focus changed dramatically and archaeologists began to ask much more of the

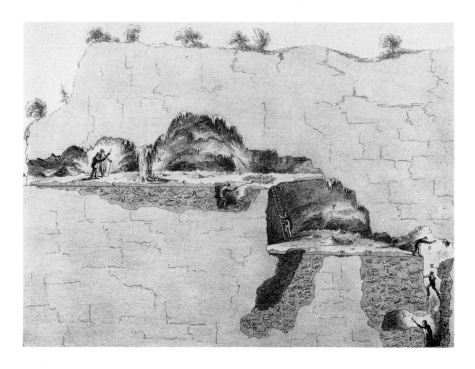

10 The excavation and study of animal bones began in the early 19th century. Dean Buckland, curator of the Museum at Oxford University, was one of the earliest academics to follow this discipline and himself excavated a number of caves. He published an account of some of his work in *Reliquiae Diluvianae* in 1823, from which this illustration is taken.

faunal remains than merely the animal species and their size. Excavations by Grahame Clark at Star Carr, England, were published in 1954. This was an exceptionally important Mesolithic site with well-preserved animal bone. Clark's association with anthropologists and palaeoecologists at Cambridge University led him to consider the significance of the faunal remains in new ways, looking at evidence for the season and character of occupation.

In the 1960s major methodological advances were made, and during this decade and the 1970s two major areas of interest developed: the evidence for early hominids in Africa, and the study of the origins of agriculture and animal husbandry. The early hominid sites in East Africa investigated by Louis Leakey and others raised questions about hominid–animal relations in the early Pleistocene and led to the adoption of taphonomy, the study of how bones become incorporated into sediments and fossilised. Developed by palaeontologists, taphonomy is used by archaeologists to understand the processes by which these sites with early hominids were formed. The big question was whether the bones of animals associated with the hominid evidence had been collected by natural agencies, by the animals or by the hominids. The origins of agriculture also became a major area for research in the 1960s, and researchers converged on the Middle East, where some of the earliest civilisations are recorded, to discover evidence for the earliest domestication of animals. Since then the subject has continued to advance and grow, and a considerable volume of work has been published all over the world.

The raw material

Today's mechanised society has systems for dealing with waste: we put it in refuse bins from which it is emptied into the back of a truck, dumped and compressed in a landfill site, and finally buried beneath soil which is then landscaped and planted. The gases generated underground as the rubbish decomposes may even be tapped and used to drive turbines that generate electricity. The 'social history' of our societies is buried beneath those green landscaped mounds as surely as it is archived in the libraries of the world. This waste may even give a 'truer' reflection of our societies – and survive longer – than the library books or the many other modern media that now record our written and visual history.

Humans in the past disposed of their waste in a less organised fashion. Since the very earliest hominids walked the earth, one of the major components of this rubbish (less varied than ours) has been the bones of animals. Initially the result of hunting or scavenging, and later of domestic animal husbandry, these bones were thrown aside, dumped in pits, floors or fires, and over time became covered and buried within the archaeological layers. Archaeologists have recognised that, in much the same way as our own garbage reflects many aspects of our culture (personal preferences, religion, status and wealth), so this material, when found and excavated, helps to illuminate the cultures of past peoples and societies. Modern landfill sites, of course, serve as communal dumps for thousands of people, whereas the animal bones that survive on archaeological sites usually reflect a much more local picture.

Preservation or survival

Many practical and analytical problems, however, make understanding the past through animal bones both complex and difficult. For a start, many factors affect the survival of animal bones both before and after their burial. Material may be weathered, frost-shattered, trampled, scavenged by dogs or other animals, moved or disturbed, all of which will affect its chances of survival. Much will be destroyed even before it is buried in the soil. It is never possible to know what has been lost, although it may be possible to recognise the agents responsible for the loss.

Even after burial, destruction of the bones may continue. The acidity or alkalinity (pH) of soil varies from acid soils with a pH of 6 or less to alkaline soils with a pH of 8 or more (a pH of 7 is neutral). Bones and teeth, which are composed of mineral and organic matter, survive poorly in acid soils, where the minerals are dissolved away and the organic component is readily broken down by bacteria. In neutral or alkaline soils where the organic component is destroyed through bacterial action, the mineral fraction survives and can last relatively unaltered for thousands of years. This mineral fraction retains the shape of the bone, so that loss of the organic component does not affect the potential for most studies. In deposits with no oxygen and little water movement, bones may survive in excellent condition, even in acid soils, due to the absence of bacteria and leaching (see fig. 40). In dry, dessicated soils, or those permanently or semi-permanently frozen, bones generally survive in exceptional condition for the same reasons, although exposure to frost will cause damage.

Nevertheless much, if not all, of the animal bone may be lost from most archaeological sites on acid soils. Sometimes only the enamel of the teeth, the densest and hardest of the skeletal tissues, survives. Evidence of the bones may exist merely as a stain or trace in the soil, and in such cases there is little to be learnt. Only material that has survived in the soil is discussed below.

Excavation and recovery

Archaeological excavation is normally conducted by trowelling the soil surface with a small pointing trowel. Whenever the texture or colour of the soil changes, it is presumed to represent a different event occurring in the past. The location, extent and thickness of each recognised layer is recorded, and the layers individually numbered. During the process of trowelling, objects and artefacts are uncovered and collected by hand, and each item is then labelled with the number of the layer from which it was recovered. In this way, the bones from each layer are recovered and the location where they were found on the site is recorded. All the bones from any one layer or group of associated layers can be pooled to form a sample or assemblage. This is extremely important because, although each bone fragment is the unit from which we gain our basic information, many of the resulting interpretations and conclusions depend upon a sample or assemblage of many such fragments.

The excavation method allows a sequence of layers, a stratigraphy, to be established which represents time. The deepest archaeological layers are usually the earliest, and those closest to the modern ground surface the most recent. In this way bones collected from the deepest levels can be analysed separately from those of the most recent layers. Likewise, the spatial relationship of the archaeological deposits permits the analysis of the bones from a particular part of an excavation independently of the bones from other parts of the site, even though the groups may be from the same stratigraphic, or contemporary time, horizon.

Manual recovery during trowelling is extremely efficient when carried out by experienced excavators with plenty of time. Nevertheless, experiments have shown that while recovery of most of the bones of sheep-sized or larger animals is generally very good, the tiny bones of these animals, such as ankle and toe bones, and the bones of much smaller animals including frogs, fishes and many birds, are often missed. They may also be damaged during the trowelling because of their fragility. These smaller species are often extremely important for environmental reconstruction and economic and dietary information, so techniques have been developed which ensure their reliable recovery.

The improved recovery techniques involve sieving the soil to enable tiny fragments of flint, pottery and bone to be easily identified and extracted. The size of the mesh can be varied in relation to the items being searched for, but if small mammal and fish bones are sought then the mesh size needs to be either 1 or 2 mm. A mesh as small as this can usually only be used effectively if the soil is washed through it with water, but in some arid or sandy areas sieving can be carried out efficiently on dry soil. If the exercise is to recover the bones of large or domestic animals, then a mesh of 8 mm is normally used (fig. 11). Water-sieving can be a very time-consuming exercise, particularly if the soil is sticky clay. It is therefore almost always necessary to introduce a 'sampling strategy' – only rarely are the results of sufficient archaeological importance to warrant the wet-sieving of all the excavated soil.

The most typical strategies used are the washing of a proportion or a fixed volume of all layers, such as 10 per cent or 25 litres, or the selection of particular

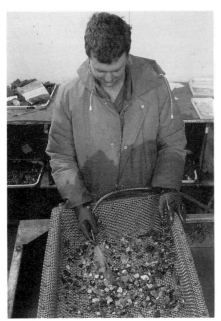

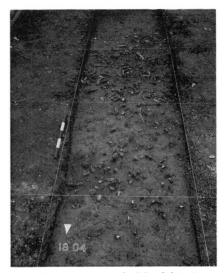

11 Not only are bones collected by hand during excavation, but various apparatuses have also been designed to sieve the excavated soil in order to improve the recovery of bones and other small finds. The simplest is washing soil through a mesh of 8mm or more to collect unbiased samples of domestic animal bones. Smaller meshes (1 or 2mm) can be used for fish bones and small rodent remains.

12 In this excavation of a Mesolithic site at Uxbridge, west London, the flints and larger bone fragments (over 5cm) were recorded three-dimensionally, as the excavation removed spits (arbitrary horizontal layers) of 5-cm depth. Each square metre of each spit was photographed. This information enables the distribution of all the bones to be reconstructed after identification. The spatial relationship of fragments of the same bone or bones from the same animal can then be determined and interpreted in terms of human activity or burial processes.

deposits, normally on the basis of their type, i.e. pit fills, floor layers, cesspits or rubbish dumps. Under the latter strategy the selection may vary considerably depending upon the character of the site and the questions that are asked about it. Questions concerning diet may concentrate on rubbish dumps and the contents of pits, while those concerning the reconstruction of the local environment may specifically sample natural sediments rather than man-made layers. Understanding changing climates through a sequence of cave deposits may require a series of samples taken vertically through the deposits. In contrast, to interpret different activities across a site, the bones from a selected number of contemporary pit fills or layers might be studied.

Although bones from each layer are generally kept separate, occasionally a greater level of detail is required. This is particularly true of questions concerning human behaviour or treatment of bone (e.g. butchery methods), or how particular deposits formed. On such occasions it is the practice to record each piece of bone identified during excavation three-dimensionally (fig. 12), and sometimes even its orientation is recorded. This is normally restricted to fragments larger than 3 or 5 cm, but can be applied to even smaller fragments. This method of recording allows the precise spatial relationships of all the bones to be reconstructed and used in the analysis, which is particularly important where fragments of the same bone, or bones of the same animal, are recovered within one or a small number of adjacent layers.

Analysis

The need for pooling the data from a number of bone fragments has already been mentioned. In order to use this information correctly it is essential that we are aware of the relationship between the fragments we have pooled to produce it. This can operate at an enormous number of levels. Bones next to each other may be presumed to have been deposited at about the same time and possibly for the same reason. An analogy might be the contents of your refuse bin the last time it was collected. Bones from a number of layers in the same pit can be assumed to represent a number of events, but probably derive from the same place or household – perhaps the contents of your refuse bin over a period of two or three months. Bones from a number of layers across an archaeological site which contain pottery of the same date are presumed to have been deposited at roughly the same time, although perhaps from a number of different sources. This might correspond to the refuse generated by your whole street and the shop on the corner over a period of one or two years. All the bones from the medieval levels of a whole site might compare with the refuse generated this century in your entire neighbourhood. The comparison is not based on the quantity generated so much as the time and variety.

It should be clear that each of these levels of information answers different questions and that each succeeding level has a much larger and more heterogeneous sample from which to draw conclusions. We learn about you (in comparison with the people living next door) from your refuse, about your street (by comparison with other streets) from its refuse, and about your neighbourhood in the twentieth century by comparison with the refuse from your own or other neighbourhoods in preceding centuries.

The relationship of layers and thereby the bones from them is fundamental to the analysis, which relies entirely on the archaeological recording of layer relationships. These layer groupings determine both the nature of the questions and the possible answers.

Analysis can be taken beyond the individual site. Bones of a particular period from many sites in one area may be the analytical unit, or even – in the case of the study of faunal changes during the Ice Ages (see fig. 16) – all the bones from sites of a particular period across a whole country.

Disturbance of buried deposits

The fact that the analysis and interpretation of animal bones generally necessitates the amalgamation of data from a number of bones introduces one of the most significant problems for studies of this type. Whereas pottery, coins and other artefacts are often intrinsically datable, there is nothing about the shape or character of a bone to say how old it is archaeologically. Radiocarbon dating using the radioactive carbon-14 isotope (half-life 5730 years) in the bone proteins may permit an assessment of the bone's age to within a hundred years or so, but this is relatively expensive and cannot be applied to more than a few key specimens.

Bone in the right burial conditions survives well and might be dug up many years later and become incorporated into layers of much younger origin. On sites with a long archaeological history, such as large towns or cities, this is a frequent problem. Natural agencies may also erode ancient deposits and move bones to new locations, where they may become buried in sediments formed many hundreds or thousands of years after the original deposition of the bone.

This process of redeposition can be recognised in the case of datable artefacts, but cannot be so easily identified from bones. It is obviously of great importance to the interpretation, which will be incorrect if the sample includes a mixture of material from completely different sources or periods.

The bone analyst therefore relies on other archaeological specialists to identify whether the sample contains only contemporary material, with little or none derived from earlier deposits. If this requirement cannot be met, then the usefulness of the sample is very limited and only the most general statements can be made. If the accompanying artefacts that can be dated intrinsically are consistent, then the analysis of the bone is considered worthwhile. However, the purity of a sample can rarely be categorically guaranteed.

Taphonomy

Much of the zoo-archaeologist's efforts are concerned with understanding how and why the bones arrived in the archaeological deposits. The study of this process was given the name taphonomy by a Russian palaeontologist trying to understand why fossils survived in rocks; it is defined as the study of the mechanisms or processes by which material moves from the biosphere (i.e. alive) to the lithosphere (i.e. fossil).

The process starts with a live animal which is hunted and slaughtered, or which may have died of natural causes such as disease. Depending on the time and place, the resulting carcass may undergo many processes. It may be scavenged or skinned and butchered by humans. The bones may be left where the animal died, or it may be jointed, carried to a camp, and distributed or sold. Not all the bones will suffer the same fate. Some may be discarded immediately, some might be carried off attached to the hide, others might be smashed immediately to extract the marrow, and yet others transported with the meat still attached.

Many alternative routes or models might be proposed. In the 'human' context these depend on the case in question, which can vary widely – from an early hominid scavenging a lion kill in southern Africa to a colonial settler slaughtering a domestic sheep in Williamsburg, Virginia, in the US. Each archaeological site is unique.

It is also important to realise that, while archaeologists are mainly concerned with human activity, they study bones from a wide variety of situations, and many different agencies may have been responsible for the accumulations.

We should consider briefly these accumulating and depositional mechanisms. Often natural agencies are responsible. Bones or carcasses are carried by water in floods and rivers and deposited when the current diminishes. Many river gravels contain the bones of animals transported during floods associated with thawing in the spring and summer during cold or glacial periods. Animals may become bogged down in marshes or other situations: examples are the marsh deposits and tar pits of Rancho Le Brea (USA) and Starunia (Poland) where, over a long period, many animals became stuck and were later preserved as a fossil assemblage. Cave sites are classic locations for prehistoric humans, but also for carnivores such as wolves, bears and hyaenas, which also accumulate bones. There are many natural traps: large animals may fall into caves or into swallow holes (water-formed holes in limestone) and small animals into pits or fissures from which they cannot extricate themselves. Some of the most dramatic bone accumulations are those resulting from people driving animals over cliffs, or into traps where large numbers are killed. The horse drives during the last glacial period in France and the killing of bison at a number of prehistoric kill sites in North America are good examples of such events.

Many of the collections of small mammal and other vertebrate bones which have proved so important for the reconstruction of climates and environments have accumulated through the actions of birds of prey. Raptors, such as eagles, hawks and particularly owls, hunt the small vertebrates of an area. The prey is eaten whole and the bones and fur later regurgitated in a pellet, which is often coughed up at special perching locations. This behaviour can result in large collections of bones building up beneath perches in locations such as cliffs, caves or wells.

However, on most occasions the agency of accumulation is human, and the majority of these accumulations are in, or close to, human habitation. The character and reason for the accumulation is often one of the objectives of the study.

Advances are continually being made in the methodology and statistics used in bone studies, permitting the reappraisal of previous work and the application of existing techniques to new areas of study. New computer-based statistical techniques can search data for patterns that would be too laborious to identify by other means. Work such as that carried out at Waterlooplein in Amsterdam, and at Pincevent and Verberie in the Paris Basin (see chapters 4 and 5), offers many possibilities for studying past activity areas and relationships between groups of people or households. Each new excavation has the potential for expanding our knowledge. Perhaps we should be looking at the bone assemblages as evidence of cultural affiliation or religious creed. Much more work is needed on the interpretation of individual groups of bone, such as might be found in pits or on floors, which would supplement the usual concentration on whole site assemblages.

— 3 —

Ecology, Climate and Time

Many of our insights into the past, and the conclusions we draw from the pieces of bone we find, are derived from our present-day understanding of animals, their ecology and distribution.

Ecology

Zoologists have recognised that particular animals occur in specific habitats, and that many of these habitats are home to a suite of species that together make up an ecological community. Although many species may be found in more than one habitat, the full suite of associated species and their relative abundance is generally typical of one particular habitat. The English fieldmouse is more typical of ground with good cover and reaches higher densities in woodland or scrub than it does on grassland. In contrast, the field vole, although found distributed over most of the English countryside, reaches its highest densities on grasslands. Roe deer are restricted to areas with either continuous or dispersed woodland, as are red deer, although in some areas this latter species is now found on moors and uplands, where they fail to attain the size typical of individuals living in deciduous forests.

These modern ecological data are extremely useful to the archaeologist interpreting animal bones. The identification of particular species at a site can be an important tool for establishing aspects of the surrounding landscape at the time. In South Africa marked changes in habitat are reflected in the faunas from Boomplaas Cave, Nelson Bay Cave and other sites. These show that the region changed, between 12,000 and 8000 years ago, from a grassland or savannah, with species such as wildebeest, hartebeest, springbok and zebra among the animals hunted by prehistoric people, to a bush and woodland habitat, reflected by the bones of bush bucks, bush pigs, buffaloes, kudus, impalas and baboons in the samples. During a similar period in Belgium, the small mammal faunas from a number of cave sites (fig. **13**) show changes in species composition and abundance that are environmentally determined. These fluctuations move from species characteristic of polar or cold, dry continental habitats to those indicative of temperate open land, such as steppe, and back again. They finally end in an increase in species related to temperate woodland.

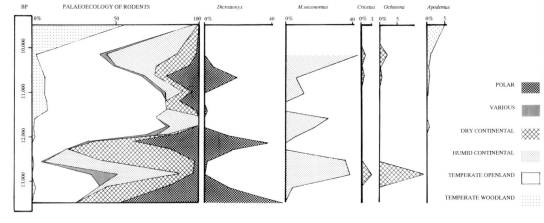

13 The mammal bones from a number of dated cave deposits in Belgium show a pattern of faunal change that reflects both climate and habitat. The arctic lemming, *Dicrostonyx torquatus*, indicates polar or tundra conditions; the northern vole, *Microtus oeconomus*, is found in humid northern coniferous forests; the steppe pika, *Ochotona pusilla*, and hamster, *Cricetus cricetus*, suggest a dry continental climate and open grasslands; and the wood mouse, *Apodemus sylvaticus*, a temperate climate and woodlands. These fluctuations reflect the major climatic changes taking place at the end of the last glaciation. (BP = years Before Present)

A temperate period may also be represented by an increase in the number, or diversity, of the species. This latter factor has been used to suggest that the local environment was wooded at the time early hominids occupied the Olduvai area of Tanzania. This site lies in the Serengeti, whose grasslands at the present are inhabited by nine species of rodent. Grasslands with lakeside woodlands in the region have eleven species, and the mixed woodland and bush of the Serengeti carries fourteen species. The fossil assemblage from Olduvai contains the remains – thought to derive from carnivore scats (droppings) – of twelve species of rodent. Carnivores are selective of prey and this suggests that not all the available rodents are present in the fossil fauna. Increasing species diversity in woodland as against open habitats is a well-recognised ecological pattern, and this high diversity at Olduvai is suggestive of a wooded rather than open habitat. Where species are extinct and their natural habitat unknown, this may be the only way of assessing the palaeoecology.

Differences in more recent environments are illustrated by the small vertebrate faunas from five sites in Britain (fig. **14**). The oldest, a Bronze Age site at Birsay, Orkney, shows a typical grassland fauna dominated by the common vole. The species from a deep well (which acted as a 'pitfall trap') at a Roman villa at Droitwich, Shropshire, is characteristic of rough grassland or wasteland, with good cover, but with some woodland nearby. In contrast, the samples from Coppergate, York, and Barnard Castle, County Durham, are dominated by species of mouse or rat, pests normally associated with humans and typical of 'urban' environments. The relative absence of more typical wild species from these two sites suggests a lack of grassland or extensive areas of waste ground. The contrast with the last site, Greyfriars, in central London, is interesting, suggesting that the gardens of the convent were extensive and contained a variety of habitats including thick grassland, scrub (perhaps shrubberies) and ditches or ponds.

	Birsay	Droitwich	Coppergate	Barnard Castle	Greyfriars Garden
	(Bronze Age)	(Roman)	(11th–13th C.)	(15th C.)	(c. 1500)
Common vole	30				
Field vole		78		1	3
Bank vole					2
Harvest mouse		1			
Common shrew		12		1	7
Pygmy shrew					5
Water shrew					7
Wood mouse	2	3			13
Water vole		13			1
Weasel		1		1	1
Pine marten		1			
Mole		3	1		
Grass snake		1			
Frog		x	6		6
Hedgehog			1		1
Red squirrel			3		
Black rat			8	3	6
House mouse			10	11	17
Hare			13	1	
Rabbit				1	

x = present but not counted

14 The number of individuals of each species identified among the bones found at five sites in Britain, from samples sieved on a mesh of either 1 or 2 mm. The common vole and the field vole are typical of grasslands, as is the mole. Common shrews are found in grassland with good cover, and the harvest mouse in long grasses and cereals. The pine marten occupies woodlands and the wood mouse and bank vole woods and hedgerows or ground with good cover. The black rat and house mouse are found in association with human habitation. The hare and rabbit were food items. The diversity of species from the garden well in the Greyfriars convent in the heart of Tudor London illustrates the richness of this artificial habitat.

Climate

Many of the differences in habitat seen above also reflect or are caused by changes in climate. The rodents from caves in Belgium (fig. **13**) show a clear progression of climatic change during the end of the last glaciation. Wild animal ranges today reflect the spatial distribution of different habitat types. Each species has evolved physiological and behavioural adaptations to particular environments. In these environments the species is relatively successful, but outside them it may be unable to survive. The ecology of each species determines its potential distribution.

Northern arctic habitats are characterised by polar bears, bearded seals, musk oxen, reindeer, arctic foxes, lemmings and arctic hares occurring in treeless tundra environments. Other northern species of less extreme range, such as the elk, wolverine and sable, are found in northern forests. Typical European temperate zone animals include the red deer, roe deer, wild boar, brown hare, wood mouse and field vole. In Mediterranean regions new species are found, including the pond tortoise and crested porcupine. Gazelles become common in the Middle East and the African faunas show a series of species shifts as habitats changed across the continent.

Age/years BC/AD	British geological divisions	Climate episodes in Britain	Industry/Period	British sites	Other sites	Age/years BC/AD
1.5 million					Olduvai Gorge, Tanzania	1.5 million
1.0 million						1.0 million
500,000	Cromerian Anglian	Interglacial Glacial				
250,000	Hoxnian	Interglacial	Clactonian Acheulian			
	Wolstonian	Glacial				
100,000	Ipswichian Devensian	Interglacial Glacial	Levalloisian	Kirkdale Cave		
50,000			Mousterian			50,000
	Upton Warren	Interstadial		Brixham Cave Isleworth		
25,000			Upper Palaeolithic		Klasies River Mouth Nelson Bay Cave Boomplaas Cave Potsdam-Schlaatz	25,000
	Windemere Loch Lomond	Interstadial Stadial	Magdalenian		Meiendorf	
10,000	Flandrian	Interglacial	Ahrensburgian		Verberie, Pincevent Stellmoor, Isturitz Ein Mallah Bedburg-Konigshoven	10,000
			Mesolithic	Uxbridge Star Carr	Ganj Dareh Tybrind Vig Mehrgarh	
5000					Çatal Hüyük Telarmachay	5000
			Neolithic			
2500					Kerma	2500
			Bronze Age	Grimes Graves Birsay, Orkney		
1000				Holloway Lane, London		1000
500 BC			Iron Age	Danebury		500 BC
0			Roman	Uley Castle Street, Carlisle Exeter Droitwich	Zwammerdam Augst	0
500 AD			Saxon	Southampton Fishergate, York		500 AD
1000 AD			Medieval	Coppergate, Aldwark, York Westminster Abbey Earls Bu and Birsay, Orkney Middlegate, Hartlepool Freswick Barnard Castle	Garnsey	1000 AD
1500 AD			Post-medieval	Greyfriars, London	Great Zimbabwe Manekweni Waterlooplein Spitzbergen Vore	1500 AD
1700 AD				Walmgate, York		1700 AD

15 This table illustrates the time periods, geological stages, climate and human industries or archaeological periods referred to in the text, and shows the approximate position on this timescale of the individual sites mentioned.

These patterns of arctic, temperate and tropical climates with tundra, deciduous forest, rain forest and savannah habitats are now the controlling influence on the distribution of individual species.

At Kirkdale Cave, in 1822, Dean Buckland found the bones of hyaenas, straight-tusked elephants, hippopotamuses and a rhinoceros, among other animals. These were all species unknown in Europe, let alone England, at the time. Since then, numerous fossil sites all over the world have yielded bones of animals either extinct or no longer found in the area. Beneath the buildings of London, the gravels, sands and silts deposited by the River Thames over the last half a million years have produced bones of hippopotamuses, lions, bison, straight-tusked elephants, woolly mammoths, fallow deer, reindeer, musk oxen, wolves, lemmings, a saiga antelope, bears and woolly rhinoceroses, to name but a few. These represent habitats as cold as the tundra and as warm as tropical Africa, and these species could not possibly all have co-existed.

It is the relationship of fauna to climate that allows the interpretation of these fossil assemblages. The association of animal bones with particular geological deposits was one of the primary methods by which the sequence of glacial and interglacial episodes of the Ice Age (fig. 15) was established in the northern hemisphere. Geologists, palaeontologists and archaeologists have all contributed to piece together the environmental and human history of this period.

Many of the species identified and named by palaeontologists are now extinct. It is often only the association in a fauna (i.e. bones of a straight-tusked elephant with a hippopotamus, or a woolly mammoth with reindeer) which allows the habitat of these extinct species to be determined.

Time

The study of faunal changes, including species extinctions, in response to climate is one of the simplest in terms of interpretation. The important information to establish is which species of animals are present, when they occur, and how these reflect the ecology and environment. The identification of all the species present in an assemblage and their relative abundance are the primary data. Changes in the species present can then be mapped on the basis of occurrences in a sequence of deposits at a single site, or through the geological correlation of the stratigraphy of a number of different sites.

This pattern of faunal change is clearly illustrated by finds of mammal species from Britain whose occurrence fluctuates with the cycle of glacial and interglacial changes (fig. 16). Through time a number of species became extinct. The recognition of those species permits not only the interpretation of cold or warm conditions, but may allow a date to be put upon the deposits, since a geological and biological stratigraphy (sequence of deposits) has been worked out over many years, and the names given to the stages usually indicate where the deposits of that date are most common or were first described.

Figures 13 and 16 also illustrate extinctions. Lemmings become locally extinct in Belgium at the top of figure 13, about 9000 years ago. In figure 16 there are three species of rhinoceros associated with the interglacial episodes: *Rhinoceros etruscus*, *R. kirchbergensis*, and *R. hemitoechus*. All were extinct by the last glaciation, but the Etruscan rhinoceros became extinct in the Cromerian/Anglian; both *R. hemitoechus* and *R. kirchbergensis* first appeared in the Hoxnian, and the latter was extinct in Britain by the Ipswichian interglacial. This sequence,

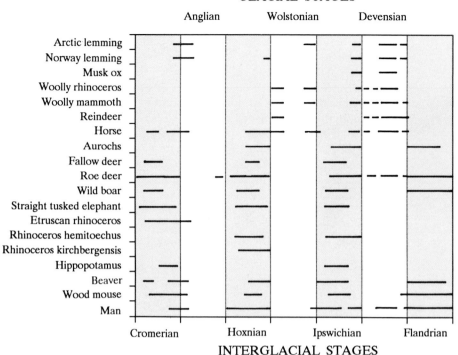

GLACIAL STAGES

Anglian   Wolstonian   Devensian

Arctic lemming
Norway lemming
Musk ox
Woolly rhinoceros
Woolly mammoth
Reindeer
Horse
Aurochs
Fallow deer
Roe deer
Wild boar
Straight tusked elephant
Etruscan rhinoceros
Rhinoceros hemitoechus
Rhinoceros kirchbergensis
Hippopotamus
Beaver
Wood mouse
Man

Cromerian   Hoxnian   Ipswichian   Flandrian

INTERGLACIAL STAGES

16 The distribution of mammal species throughout the Ice Age clearly shows the alternate changes from a warm (interglacial) fauna to a cold (glacial) fauna. A selection of species from the Pleistocene of Britain are here arranged with the cold-habitat animals at the top, and those associated with warm climates below. The bars indicate the presence of dated remains (the timescale is not linear). The Arctic species are found in deposits that date to the very beginning or end of the interglacials, as the climate is changing, and during the glacial episodes. Many of the warm-climate species are only found in the middle (or warmest) part of the interglacials.

developed from the faunas of a number of sites, can be used to age the deposits in which the bones occur. Finds of Etruscan rhinoceros would indicate a faunal assemblage of Cromerian age, while that of *R. kirchbergensis* would show the deposits were of Hoxnian interglacial date.

The use of faunal remains to show these time and climate episodes has largely been overtaken by isotope studies on deep-sea sediments and cores of the polar ice, which show fluctuations in the temperature in the northern hemisphere over the last two million years, but they may still be important for dating local sequences of deposits.

Although these faunal changes are normally analysed at one locality or region, it is important to realise that they represent the movement of animals into and out of the region. As the glaciers of the northern hemisphere advanced and the ice sheets moved south, the arctic animals were pushed south into previously temperate areas. The temperate species were themselves pushed south into the Mediterranean region, and so on. During a warm or interglacial period the sequence of movement is reversed, although extinctions may have occurred or species may never have returned to their former range.

Movement and migration

These movements on a grand scale are predicted from the faunas of many sites whose age is known from geological and other means, but much smaller-scale seasonal movements of animals can also be established from bone studies. Many of the animals hunted by early humans, particularly in Europe, were migratory, and moved on a seasonal round from summer calving grounds to winter grazing. Reindeer present in central England 40,000 years ago spent only their winters in this area, a pattern indicated by the presence of shed antlers of male animals only in many river deposits of this period. Modern male caribou and reindeer shed their antlers in late winter after the rut, while females retain them until after the summer calving. These populations must have moved some distance to their summer grounds, probably north or out on to the plains now covered by the North Sea. In contrast, the bison whose remains occur in the same deposits spent their summers in central England and probably moved south and east on to the dry or marshy North Sea basin or crossed over to northern France during the winter to escape the cold.

Studies on the reindeer assemblages from central France (fig. 17) have enabled the probable migration routes of certain populations to be predicted. The evidence from the seasonal hunting of this species by the Magdalenian hunters of ten to fifteen thousand years ago, together with our knowledge of the ecology and migration patterns of modern reindeer and caribou and the ability to date the sites, have suggested the winter grazing and summer calving grounds for a number of populations in France and Belgium.

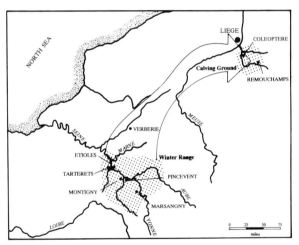

17 The probable migration route of reindeer found in the winter on the Magdalenian sites in the Paris Basin and in the summer at calving grounds near Liège. A number of such migrations have been postulated in France and Belgium. The time of year that reindeer are present at a site is determined from the age structure of the sample, the presence of antlers at different stages of development, and studies of the tooth cementum. Where different sites can be shown to be of the same date, but with evidence of occupation at a different season, it is possible to suggest the migrational round of the reindeer.

The time span during the Ice Ages is large in human terms and the archaeological significance of animal bone collections from many deposits of this period is primarily related to understanding the geological history of the deposits and only incidentally to providing a chronological and environmental backdrop to the human fossils that are found. Towards the end of this period, however, humans exerted a much greater influence over their environment and the animal bones become more important as evidence of human actions.

— 4 —

Early Human Exploitation

Although tool-using hominids are now known to have been around for as long as one and a half to two million years, evidence for their exploitation of animals is very limited. Most of the evidence for hominids is in the stone tools they used and rare fossils of the hominids themselves.

Bones and early hominids

While it is possible to reconstruct the physical anthropology of these hominids from their own bones, the presence of tools – crude though they may be – is indicative of the ability to manipulate external objects to their advantage. It is of some importance to students of early human life to establish whether behavioural traits led to brain development, or vice versa; and whether ancient humans were omnivorous scavengers, collecting and scavenging food resources in a manner typical of modern apes, or predators actively using their capacity to make 'tools' and their ability to coordinate behaviour in order to kill prey otherwise beyond their physical capabilities. Also important is whether or not they functioned within social or family groups, sharing food resources and having definable camps where social interaction and feeding was concentrated. Apart from the tools used, the only surviving material with which to tackle these questions is the animal bones found associated with the stone tools. Archaeologists have turned their attention to these bones with, at present, only a marginal measure of success.

The simplest use of bones in this context is represented by the association of flint with bone remains (fig. 18).

Clear evidence of cut marks made by a stone implement on the bones of animals being butchered or skinned is perhaps one of the earliest indications of hominids using objects purposefully. Such evidence has now been recognised on bones from East African sites of Plio-Pleistocene age, around 1.8 million years ago (fig. 19). Other physical evidence is suggestive of tool use. Hammerstones produce what are called 'spiral' fractures of bone, and 'primitive' peoples often use such implements for breaking long bones in order to extract the rich marrow. However, such fractures can be generated naturally, and attribution of hominid

LOW	MODERATE	HIGH
Transitory camps		Kill or butchery sites
Quarry or workshop sites		Camp or occupation sites

Decreasing density of stone artefacts →

Increasing density of bone

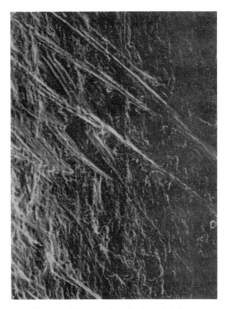

18 Differences in the distributional density of bones and stone tools are seen as an indication of site function. A clear relationship between bones and stone tools is viewed as evidence of the accumulation of the bones by hominids or humans as a result of food-procuring activities. High concentrations of bone and artefacts are thought to represent evidence of a 'base camp' or habitation area, while low densities of tools and bone would suggest a hunting site or transitory camp. (This 'model' takes no account of other possible mechanisms that might have been responsible for the bone accumulations.)

19 Clear evidence of early hominids as accumulators of bones is given where bones have cut marks made on them by stone tools. It is possible through microscopic analysis to differentiate between scratches or cuts made by stone tools and those made by accidental abrasion or animal gnawing. These scratches, photographed using a scanning electron microscope and printed at a magnification of 20x, occur on the shaft of the distal humerus of an extinct ungulate, *Kobus sigmoidalis*, over 1.5 million years old from a site in the Olduvai Gorge, Tanzania – testimony to the antiquity of tool use.

influence is therefore problematic. Polish and wear on bones have been used to suggest usage of bone fragments as tools – but even such wear can be caused by abrasion in sand and trampling by wild ungulates.

While such investigations are part of the effort to recognise evidence of tool-using hominids, they are equally important as evidence of the development of behaviour related to intellectual ability and thought. This is because a carcass yields a number of different resources for human exploitation – the skin, tendons, bone, meat and marrow – each of which demands a different treatment. Nevertheless, the marks found on bones do not answer questions as to whether the animals so butchered were hunted or scavenged.

Scavenging vs hunting

Considerable debate has been waged in the academic literature over this subject and some authors have reached opposite conclusions from the same evidence. Two theoretical approaches have been employed. One involves the analysis of the location of cut marks on identified bones in conjunction with the diversity of species represented among these bones. Where a carcass is dismembered for subsequent carrying or distribution, the cut marks would be expected to be concentrated around the joints of the major meat-bearing bones in order to divide the carcass easily. An assumption is also made that hunting is usually specialist and therefore generally concentrated on one or two species of similar habit and habitat. At Olduvai, Tanzania, between one and a half and two million years ago, cut marks were concentrated on the mid-shaft regions rather than joints, indicating no preference for meat-bearing bones. They also occurred on a wide range of species from small bovids to giraffids. This assemblage has therefore been interpreted as the result of opportunistic exploitation of carcasses for a variety of products likely to include tendons, skin and bone as well as meat. Such conclusions are used to formulate a picture of early hominids in small groups or solitary, with a scavenging and foraging mode of life and no base or camp, in contrast to the simpler model suggested in figure **18**.

The second theoretical approach utilises the distribution of the various parts of the carcass of food animals at the site to support the scavenging inference. In this argument it is presumed that the archaeological assemblage will be dominated by those bones of greatest food utility that still survive after a non-hominid predator has eaten at least part of the prey carcass. The assumptions here are that the best meat 'units' were consumed at the kill by the predator, and also that a dried, half-eaten carcass demands different butchery techniques to that of a fresh, recently killed animal. The incidence of animal gnawing indicates exploitation by animals, which may of course occur before or after hominid use. Interestingly, analyses of this sort require only recognition of the type of bone and the size and type of animal. The specific identification of which species are present is incidental. In a study carried out on a middle Stone Age cave site at Klasies River Mouth, South Africa, the presence of high counts of important meat-bearing bones of the small bovids (grysbok and other species) in the assemblage, and the very low counts of foot bones, were used to suggest that these small bovids were hunted and then dismembered at the kill site, and that the favoured units were carried back to the cave (fig. **20**). The contrasting picture for the large bovids, such

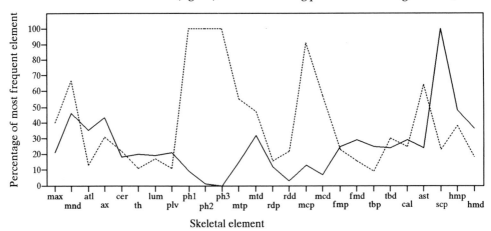

20 The frequency of occurrence of various parts of the skeleton of large and small bovids at the site of Klasies River Mouth, South Africa, varies considerably. The smaller bovids (*solid line*) show high frequencies of the major limb bone fragments (humerus, scapula, femur). These are seen as bones with high attached meat value. The large bovids (*dotted line*), in contrast, have high numbers of phalanges, metapodials and jaws – bones carrying less meat.

as Cape buffalo and eland, with high incidences of feet, lower limbs and head parts, is seen as the scavenging of exploitable parts remaining from kills already made by other predators. This was supported by the frequent evidence of tooth and gnawing marks on these bones, in contrast to those of the small bovids, and a significantly higher incidence of what are described as hack marks, thought to be the result of dismembering a dried rather than a fresh carcass.

These are simply two examples of the manner in which the recognition of bones and their attendant attributes can be used to reconstruct patterns of the past. Another analysis of the Klasies River Mouth site postulated that both large and small animals were hunted, the smaller bovids normally being transported whole to the cave site while only selected bones of the larger animals were kept. Perhaps the feet bones attached to the skins were used as handles to carry the filleted meat from the heavier limb bones, or possibly they were kept because the sinews in the feet were important for use as cords.

Human and animal accumulations

With such questions being posed, it has always been important to determine when a bone collection has been accumulated by human agency or by the activities of other animals. Many years ago Dean Buckland concluded that the bones and teeth of fossil and extinct mammals in Kirkdale Cave had accumulated through hyaena activity, based on a simple comparison with the bone debris, fractures and tooth marks of modern hyaena accumulations. A number of animals accumulate bones, in caves particularly: bears, wolves, foxes, big cats, hyaenas and even porcupines, which gnaw the bones to stop their teeth growing too long. Some of these animals have in the past competed for living space with humans and early hominids, and the juxtaposition of bear and other carnivore remains with those of humans is not uncommon in late Pleistocene caves in Europe.

The identification of which animal is responsible for the bone debris utilises methods similar to those already mentioned above. Different carnivores eat and destroy carcasses to varying extents. Hyaenas with their extremely strong jaws crush the shafts of long bones, producing characteristic splinters. Individual species may treat different prey species differently. For example, members of the cat family and their extinct relatives eat and destroy the vertebral column and sometimes the pelvis of primates such as monkeys and baboons, while leaving the much harder and angular vertebral column of ungulates such as zebras and wildebeests relatively untouched. These animals rarely fracture the long bones of bovids in the manner of hyaenas. Jawbones have a high survival potential, since the enamel of the teeth is very hard and only the margins of the bone are normally chewed. The results of hyaena activity may sometimes be very similar to the fracturing by humans of long bones for the extraction of the bone marrow, using a hammerstone and anvil. Identification of these animals as accumulators requires detailed observations of tooth and gnawing marks, patterns of bone survival, and patterns of breakage. Human evidence is most easily determined through visible cut or hack marks, and traces of burning on the bone; otherwise, external factors such as associated artefacts must be used.

Authorities tend to agree that by the time *Homo erectus* had evolved, about one and a half million years ago, and had developed the tool kit associated with the Acheulian period, humans were predatory omnivores, relying on hunted game as well as gathered foodstuffs. In many Pleistocene cave and open sites in Europe and elsewhere the association of artefacts, bones, cut marks and archaeological circumstances have been sufficient to rule out the possibility of other animals being responsible for the bones.

Specialised hunters

During the last Ice Age early humans, whether *Homo sapiens sapiens* or *Homo sapiens neanderthalensis*, became specialist hunters, as were many of the carnivores. They had a clearly developed social organisation, with communication levels sophisticated enough for developing co-operative hunting strategies. Many Upper Palaeolithic sites in central and western Europe exhibit a concentration on one major prey species, although the chosen species varies.

Reindeer are one of the most ubiquitous prey species and a common prey specialisation during the last glaciation in Europe. Many archaeological samples from the Upper Palaeolithic in France, Germany and elsewhere are dominated by the bones of this species. At the open hunting station at Stellmoor, Germany, where 656 individual animals were recognised among the bones, 650 of these were reindeer. In France many sites also have very large numbers of horse bones, indicating specialisation in the hunting of this animal. At Isturitz, in the French Basque country, the bones include large numbers of jaws which indicate animals of all ages and suggest indiscriminate hunting by mass drives, like those of the bison by North American Palaeo-Indians. Similar specialisation in horses is found from Mousterian to Magdalenian times (about 40,000 to 10,000 years ago), and from eastern through to western Europe. In the Pyrenees, Magdalenian sites on upland cliffs exhibit specialised ibex hunting where up to 90–100 per cent of the ungulate bones are ibex. The presence of ptarmigan and grouse amongst the assemblages is indicative of exploitation of one of the few other animal food resources in these upland regions. In many of the French sites in the Dordogne, salmon bones are a common find, and the absence of head bones among the remains has been used to postulate that the fish were hunted during their summer run to the spawning grounds further downstream and then dried before being carried up to these sites. Some North American Indians on the north-west coast relied heavily on these seasonal runs of salmon, as some communities still do today. Later, as the climate warmed and temperate forests spread northwards, different species became important as prey in Europe. Red deer were intensively hunted, and wild ox, elk and roe deer bones are frequently found.

Kill sites, camps and food value

It is fairly straightforward to establish which species were killed and eaten by prehistoric hunters, but the bones can tell us very much more about these events. The simplest interpretations relate to kill sites, butchery and base camps. The archaeological evidence in late Palaeolithic and Mesolithic sites is both more abundant and better preserved than early hominid sites and interpretation of the taphonomy of the assemblages is less of a problem.

As long ago as 1952 an American archaeologist, Theodore White, considered what might be left behind and what would be transported by hunters butchering a carcass at the kill site. Presumably the elements of greatest utility or food value would be carried off. Theoretically the skin, probably with feet attached, the rib

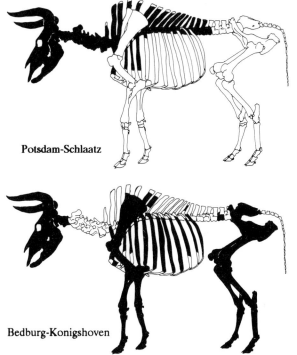

Potsdam-Schlaatz

Bedburg-Konigshoven

21 Bone survival is used to show the nature of a site. In these examples the aurochs (wild ox) from Potsdam-Schlaatz (*top*) had only its skull, vertebrae and a few ribs left on the site, a 'typical' kill site assemblage. In contrast, the remains from Bedburg-Königshoven (*bottom*), of at least six individuals, show high concentrations of limb bones, ribs and skull fragments, but very few vertebrae, an assemblage of higher utility elements indicative of a temporary hunting camp, the presence of skull fragments perhaps suggesting the animals were hunted close by.

cage and the upper limb bones would be taken away with other meat stripped from the vertebrae and rump. This would leave at the kill site the skull and vertebral column, and possibly some lower-value elements of the limbs. The demand for food resources and the number of hunters would affect the degree to which any one site might reflect the theory. Figure 21 illustrates two examples, one interpreted as a kill site and the second as butchering waste at an occupied summer camp. This theory has since been built upon by another American, Lewis Binford, who observed at Nunamiut Eskimo caribou kill sites that bones of high utility were in low frequency and those of low value in high numbers. He developed a 'General Utility Index' to take account of the value of each skeletal element in terms of its meat, marrow and fat. He further considered that some bones may – because of their attachment to elements of higher utility – be transported incidentally, and he therefore modified the index to take account of this. Each element or part of an element was given an index to measure its likelihood of removal from the kill site to a camp. This information, collected from a modern Eskimo hunting community, has been used by many researchers to analyse a number of archaeological samples (see fig. 25).

At Star Carr, a significant Mesolithic site in Yorkshire, England, occupied at about 7500 BC, the bones of red and roe deer, wild oxen, elk and wild boar have provided a series of important insights into the past. The season of occupation of the site is indicated by the evidence of the deer antlers, which develop and are shed over a known seasonal cycle; the presence of bones from a neonatal elk that died at or soon after birth in May, June or July; and the presence of many jaws from deer that must have died between May and October (fig. 22). It is clear that most of the evidence indicates that the animals were killed between April and October, and that all *could* have been killed between May and September. There

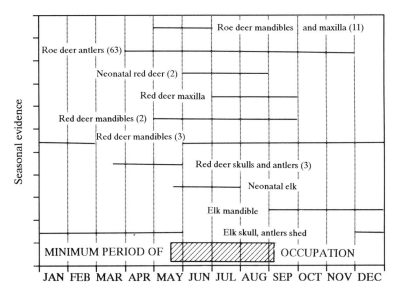

Season of death

22 *above* A number of the bones from the Mesolithic site at Star Carr indicate the season in which the animals were killed. The pattern of tooth eruption in the roe deer compares closely with that of modern animals killed in mid-May. Roe deer carry their antlers between April and November and all 63 specimens have unshed antlers. The neonatal red deer and elk are animals only a few weeks old, indicating that they died in the summer, since calving takes place in late spring or early summer. Two of the red deer skulls had shed their antlers: this takes place in late winter, indicating death between March and June.

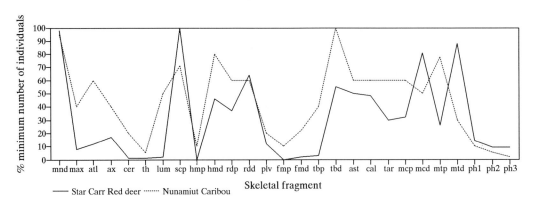

— Star Carr Red deer ······ Nunamiut Caribou   Skeletal fragment

23 The red deer bone sample from Star Carr is here compared with the bones of caribou collected from a Nunamiut Eskimo hunting camp in north central Alaska. The minimum number of animals (MNI) was estimated from the bones and the frequency of each bone as a percentage of the MNI plotted for each sample. The representation of the different parts of the carcass is very similar at both sites. By analogy, it is suggested that the Star Carr site therefore has a bone distribution pattern that is likely to be found at a hunting camp.

is no clear evidence for animals killed in winter. What type of site was this? The frequency of the individual bones of the skeleton of red deer, the most common prey animal, is not indicative of a kill site, so further comparisons were made between the archaeological sample and the Nunamiut base camp and hunting camp assemblages (fig. 23). These comparisons show a close similarity between the frequency of bones of red deer from this 9500-year-old site in Yorkshire and those of reindeer from the 1950s Eskimo hunting camp. The interpretation rests upon the acceptance of a universally similar treatment of similar-sized ungulates by hunting communities. Minor variations are seen as resulting from different cultural rather than dietary demands; loss through damage by scavenging dogs; and ease and method of transport from the kill sites to the base camps. So we can suggest that the meat element of the diet of Mesolithic people in Yorkshire was largely made up of hunted red and roe deer, wild ox and elk. The hunters occupied the site at Star Carr during the early and possibly middle summer, probably as a camp to which they returned with selected food items and hides from kill sites.

By estimating the minimum number of animals present among the bones (from the most frequently occurring element) and using modern data to suggest the potential food weight or value of the carcass of each species, it is possible to calculate the possible nutritional value of the hunted animals. This gives a total meat weight of 12,029 kg from 26 red deer, 12 elk, 16 wild oxen, 11 roe deer and 4 wild pigs. When converted into calories (on the basis of dietary figures calculated from modern venison), and assuming an average daily energy requirement of 2280 kilocalories per person, this weight of meat might supply the caloric needs of four family units (eight adults and twelve children) for nearly a year, or a six-man hunting party (with a daily intake of 3000 kilocalories) for two and a half years. These should not be seen as reconstructions but merely order-of-magnitude data which allow the inference that the site, if a summer hunting camp, might have been used for between two and three weeks each year over a period of fifty to sixty years – assuming that all the food was consumed by this party – or rather less if much of it was removed to a base camp elsewhere.

We can extend this type of interpretation even further if we consider a fifteenth-century North American bison kill site at Garnsey, New Mexico. At this site the archaeological remains represent a number of individual events at which one or a number of bison were killed and subsequently butchered. These events are thought to have been separated by a few days, weeks or at most a number of years. The bone sample comprised 6937 bison bones. The number of bison represented on the site was calculated from the most frequently occurring bone, which was the skull, and indicated at least thirty-five animals. This is a minimum estimate, since the skulls of some of the prey may have been removed. An analysis of the teeth of these animals, based on the evidence of eruption, the pattern of wear on the surface of the teeth and measurements of the height of the tooth crown (see fig. 33), established that the animals must have been killed during the spring calving season. This would be April/May on the evidence of modern northern Plains bison, or late March/April when compared with the calving time of southern Plains populations. The age structure of the bison is based upon the same dental evidence, and shows two peaks among the animals, one at three to four years of age and a second at seven. This is not a catastrophic kill pattern, when a whole herd is killed – which would include animals of all ages in the proportion they occur in the live population. Such a group would be

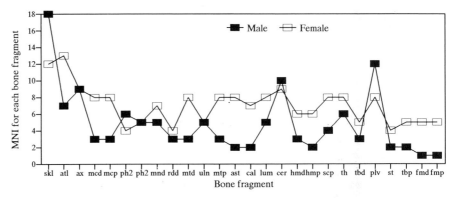

24 Measurement data was used to ascertain the sex of the bison bones from Garnsey, New Mexico. The minimum number of individuals (MNI) represented by each of these elements is plotted. It is clear that most of the bones are represented by higher frequencies of females than males, although the male skulls are the most frequent bone (18 individuals). The bones have been arranged from left to right in order of utility (MGUI), from low to high, showing a general drop in frequency at the kill site correlating with increasing value.

dominated by juveniles and young calves, with decreasing numbers of progressively older age groups.

The excavated evidence supports the archaeological inference of multiple kill events. Male and female bison are significantly different in size (see fig. **4**) and it is therefore possible to sex many of the bones using measurements. The results of these analyses are presented in graph form in figure **24**. The most frequent bone, the skull, has a sex ratio of 60:40 males to females, as does the pelvis. In contrast, the majority (73 per cent) of the non-head elements show a female domination among the bones. The analysts, having considered the reasons for these apparent biases (sampling or problems of sexing), concluded that this discrepancy was due to human behaviour. Two of the options considered for this sexual bias were that the female skulls were selectively butchered or removed from the site, or that many post-cranial bones of males were selectively removed.

There is little evidence of the butchery of skulls on site and very few skull fragments; also, the skull is viewed as a unit of very low general utility (fig. **24**) and therefore one of the most suitable elements from which to establish the sex ratio of the original killed population. This, combined with the observation that there is a strong tendency for the female bones to decrease in number with increasing general utility (fig. **24**), suggests that it is unlikely that significant numbers of female skulls have been removed, and the original killed population probably approximated to the 60:40 male/female skull ratio. While caribou and bison differ much more than caribou and red deer, the Modified General Utility Index derived from observation of the modern caribou hunters was applied to the study of the Garnsey bison in an effort to discover whether the butchering and removal of the bison bones was based upon their utility. The distribution displayed a relationship which indicated that only the lowest utility value units occurred in large numbers and that both medium- and high-value anatomical elements are missing, suggesting removal from the site with attached food re-

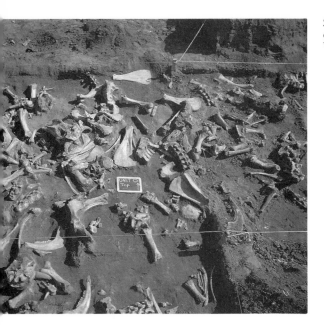

25 An example of the excavated remains of bison from a 300-year-old kill site at Vore, Wyoming, in North America.

sources. Perhaps of even more interest is that when this distribution is plotted for males and females independently (see fig. **24**), a much higher than expected proportion of the female bones survive at the site than their utility index would predict. Not only do a higher proportion of the female bones survive on site, but a much lower incidence of breakage of the major limb bones due to butchery or marrow processing is present among the discarded female elements.

These results are used to argue for a heavy discrimination against the butchery, marrow extraction and removal of female bones from the kill sites. The analyses showed that this was most marked against the metacarpal and metatarsal bones, which are important marrow bones but carry very little meat. These data can be used in conjunction with modern zoological information to give an interpretation of the behaviour of the hunters at Garnsey. At the time when these animals were killed (spring), male bison are in generally good condition and have recovered after the summer rut, during which their fat reserves are depleted due to rutting and limited feeding. Their condition improves rapidly during the late spring and early summer prior to the next rut. Females, in contrast, are in their poorest condition at this time of year because it is the calving season; they have been carrying their young and are lactating. They gradually improve throughout the summer after calving. At Garnsey the males killed would have been in good condition, although by no means peak, while the females are likely to have been in their poorest condition, with seriously depleted fat reserves.

Fats are an important part of the human diet, and the consumption within a hunting population, with no alternative fats sources, of exclusively lean meat will lead to nutritional problems. In the late winter and spring human groups are themselves likely to be under some nutritional stress, and the demand for fats, with their high calorific potential, would have been high. The bone evidence can therefore be used to suggest that, at this site, groups of bison hunted and killed in spring were then selectively butchered in response to the food needs of the human population, resulting in relatively low-intensity exploitation of the female bison in poor condition, but intense exploitation and removal of the medium- and high-value anatomical parts from the male animals to camps elsewhere on the plains. The high ratio of males, in the light of this interpretation, suggests that the hunters in spring concentrated on hunting male bison groups. The bone analysis, when combined with modern ecological data, has given us considerable insight into the behaviour, preferences and demands of this hunting group. We might expect, should we find an autumn kill, that it would show the preferential removal of the bones of females, then in good condition relative to males.

Although of relatively recent date, this fifteenth-century North American example could as easily reflect behavioural selection within an Ice Age hunting society in Europe specialising in reindeer, horse or bison.

Hunting technology

In Schleswig-Holstein, Germany, in the late glacial period, one reindeer migration route took the herds through Tunnel Valley along the Wandse River. Two very famous sites, at Meiendorf and Stellmoor, lie in this valley and excavations have yielded the remains of many reindeer. These sites date to 10,000 and 8000 BC respectively. The latter shows slaughter mainly in the autumn, prior to the rut, when the animals were in good condition. However, humans appear to have occupied the site all year round, probably utilising cached meat and stored grease and marrow fat when other food resources were scarce, much as modern caribou hunters do.

Stellmoor is particularly interesting because many of the bones from the Ahrensburgian levels exhibit hunting wounds, some with flints embedded in the bone (fig. 26). An analysis of their location and angle of entry has yielded interesting insights into the hunting practices. There is no evidence of arrows being released before the animals came abreast and exposed their whole flanks. A small group of wounds indicate shots made as the animal moved away from the hunter and, given the location of the kills at the bottom of the valley, and the angle of entry, these are consistent with shots fired at animals trying to make their escape by swimming into the lake away from the hunter. A number of the wooden shafts

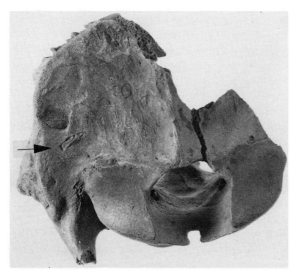

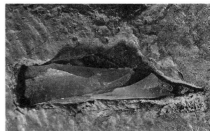

26 The tip of a flint arrow head has become embedded in the rear of the skull of a reindeer. The shot must have been fired as the animal moved away from the hunter. This specimen comes from Ahrensburgian levels at Stellmoor, Schleswig-Holstein, Germany.

from the arrows were found in the lake muds. No doubt traps and spears took their toll, but only arrow damage has been found on the bones.

Activity areas

We have briefly considered some of the information to be gained from whole sites, but it is also possible from the distribution and analysis of the bones to make interpretations of functional areas within a site and aspects of the communal sharing of food resources. An important excavation at Verberie in the Paris Basin, which dates to the Magdalenian period and, like other contemporary sites, represents a specialist reindeer hunting group, has produced some of the earliest evidence for activity areas within a site. The distribution of bone fragments and flints is shown in figure 27, and the areas with no bone or flint are clearly distinguishable. The distribution of waste bones associated with the initial butchering of a carcass, such as the vertebrae, tail and metapodials, are grouped around these empty areas, suggesting that the animal being dismembered occupied this space. Other bones are found elsewhere on the camp or near a hearth, and certain areas distinguished by flint blades believed to be used for cutting meat suggest an area in which further processing of the food took place. At Pincevent, a site of similar date in the Paris Basin, the bones of different parts of the same individual are found at more than one hearth. These are identified by the refitting of fragmented bones or articulations, like a jigsaw, or by the matching of left and right parts – which is relatively easy if fragmentation is not too severe and the number of individuals is small. The bones of nine different individuals were found shared between three separate hearths. These hearths were between 6 and 10 metres apart, a sufficient distance to suggest that such finds are not accidental, and do not represent the post-consumption movement of the bones. We have come one and a half million years from the hypothesised food-sharing of early hominids in East Africa before relatively conclusive proof of food-sharing can be deduced from animal bones.

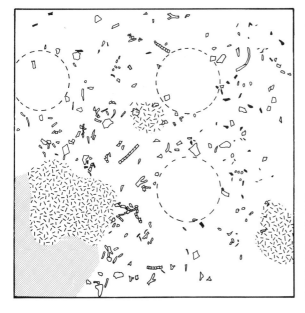

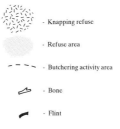

- Knapping refuse

- Refuse area

- Butchering activity area

- Bone

- Flint

27 The distribution of bones at Verberie in the Paris Basin suggests the areas of the site where the carcasses of reindeer were being butchered. The absence of bones and flint tools in particular patches is believed to represent the position in which the carcass itself lay. Sequences of vertebrae, bones rejected early during butchery, can be seen around these areas.

— 5 —

Domestication, Husbandry and Food

Nearly ten thousand years ago, while Europe and most other parts of the world were still inhabited by hunting peoples, a revolution was taking place in an area of the Middle East known as the Fertile Crescent, from Turkey through Iraq to Iran along the valleys of the Tigris and Euphrates rivers. This revolution was the domestication of plants and animals. The resulting control of food resources, both plant and animal, within a defined area and without the necessity of hunting, led to a major change in the cultural development of humans. It is often said that this area saw the birth of civilisation as we know it. Confirmation of the existence of domestication has been a major objective of academic research in the Middle East, and over the last three decades the dating of the earliest evidence for domestic animals and plants has been pushed backwards, with domestic dogs now recognised from about 10,000 BC and the first domestic goats and sheep from about 7000 BC. Although independent archaeological evidence for the presence of domestic animals is also available from other finds, it is the analyses of the bones themselves that form the major body of evidence.

Domestication

The criteria by which domestication in animals is recognised are as follows, although there is some argument about their reliability:

- the presence of a species at a site outside the known natural distribution of this species in the wild;
- a marked change in species exploitation from one archaeological level to the next, where the more recent level shows a high proportion of species now domesticated;
- a noticeable change in the age structure of the killed animals, which might be interpreted as deriving from a controlled herd rather than hunted wild groups;
- a change in the sex ratio within the bones that can be sexed, suggesting preferential selection of a sex category, likely to be possible only if the animals are being herded;
- a marked decrease in size or a change in bone shape from earlier or contemporary known wild individuals of the species.

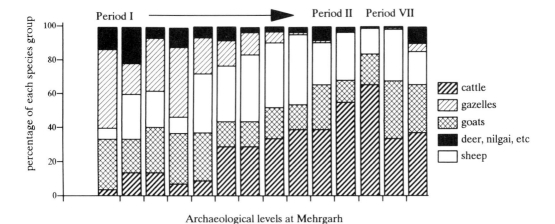

Archaeological levels at Mehrgarh

28 The faunal remains from Mehrgarh date to the 8th millennium BC in the earliest levels (**I**). During the next millennium (**II**) the spectrum of species changes, from one dominated by deer and gazelles to the dominance of cattle, sheep and goats, almost to the exclusion of the gazelles and deer, a pattern still present in the 3rd millennium (**VII**). This change is seen as evidence for the cattle having been domesticated in the later levels, illustrating a move from a hunting community in the earliest levels to a society relying heavily on domestic animals.

The first criterion, the appearance of a species outside its wild range, is of little interest to students studying the 'earliest' domestication since (for obvious reasons) this always takes place within the wild animal's range. On the other hand, domestic animals appear at different times in the archaeological record across the world as they are introduced already domesticated from elsewhere. In Britain the wild sheep, or mouflon, the progenitor of our domestic sheep, does not occur naturally and never has, so early finds of sheep (and for that matter goats) can immediately be taken as domestic animals. Such a conclusion is much more difficult for cattle, whose wild ancestor the aurochs (*Bos primigenius*) is native to Britain and continued to survive in the wild for possibly two thousand years after the earliest identified bones of domestic cattle.

At Mehrgarh in Baluchistan, in south-western Pakistan, the faunal sequence in the archaeological deposits spans from the fifth to the seventh millennium BC and illustrates well the second criterion (fig. 28). There is a decreasing proportion of definite wild species, such as gazelle, deer and nilgai, while the proportions of cattle bones rise. The latter are therefore seen as domestic in the later levels. Interestingly, the goat and sheep bones show no such convincing pattern, even though the site lies within the range of the wild species. It is therefore not clear when domestic animals become more important than their wild cousins, although the goats show a decrease in size (the fifth criterion) before the cattle numbers rise, suggesting that domestic goats occurred earlier at the site than cattle.

In the Levant and Anatolia the change from gazelles, the major prey species for hunters 10,000 years ago, to species now domesticated is found on a number of sites, where they are normally replaced first by goat bones, with those of sheep becoming more abundant a little later. In these instances it is useful not just to examine the different layers of a single site but to see if the patterns are reflected in a group of sites of overlapping periods in the same geographical area.

Some changes in the age structure of the bone samples are thought to show changes from hunting to the controlled exploitation of hitherto wild ungulates. Low numbers of the bones of neonates (stillborn or very recently born animals) are expected in a sample deriving from a hunted population. The return on such young animals is small, and hunting preference for pregnant or lactating females might be unlikely due to their poor condition. However, a herd of animals controlled by pastoralists generally involves newborn animals being closely looked after near the focus of human habitation, and deaths from a variety of causes are likely to produce a concentration of the bones of such animals in the settlement.

This argument has been used to interpret a change from hunting to the herding of goats on a number of sites in the Middle East and the domestication of llama and alpaca from the wild camelids in South America (fig. **29**). At the site of Ganj Dareh in the Zagros Mountains, in Iran, a combination of sex and age estimates on the bones of goats showed a pronounced pattern. In the early levels

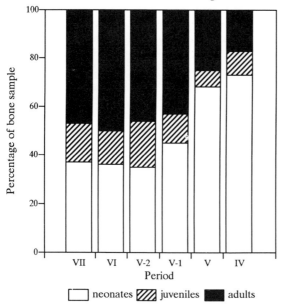

29 The camelidae (guanaco and vicuna) at Telarmachay, Peru, show a marked increase in the number of neonatal bones on the site after period V-2 (4800–4000 BC). This is consistent with one of the criteria for domestication, an increase in neonates on the site, indicating control of a breeding population. This change was accompanied by some specimens with a dental morphology typical of modern domestic llama and alpaca.

30 *below* The goat metatarsals from Ganj Dareh, in west central Iran, were measured to study sexual dimorphism. Both adult and immature specimens were measured. The immature specimens are generally larger than the mature ones and the distribution suggests two groups. These are interpreted as males and females. The data also shows that most of the males are immature while most of the females are mature.

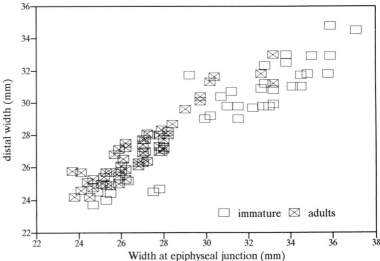

at this site, data derived from tooth eruption, epiphyseal fusion and bone measurements show a dramatic difference in the selection of males and females of different ages (fig. 30); and although the original author interprets this as reflecting the hunting of nursery herds of wild goat (females with kids and immature males), it could equally be interpreted as the preferential slaughter of young males for meat and the retention of females for breeding and milk. This is a good example of the contradictory conclusions that can be drawn from the same osteological data, and reveals the problems that beset the recognition of domestication.

Domestication is believed to lead generally to a discernible decrease in the size of animals. It is true that, on many excavations in the Middle East and Europe dating to these early periods, such a size decrease is clearly visible. This does not, however, allow us to predict the wild or domestic character of an individual specimen. A recent review of Middle Eastern cattle neatly illustrates these size changes (fig. 31). The evidence suggests that the cattle of the Near East are not clearly domestic until the sixth millennium BC.

The development of pastoralism alongside animal domestication introduces a whole new series of questions for the zoo-archaeologist, and for this period onwards a large volume of work has been published. A few selected examples will show how the data collected from the bones aid our understanding of more recent periods.

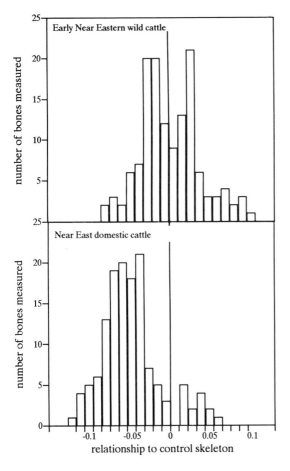

31 When bone samples are small, such as for cattle from early Near Eastern sites, it is often impossible to obtain a large enough sample of a single bone to study size changes. This can be rectified by measuring the bones of a single skeleton (in this case a female Danish aurochs) and plotting each archaeological bone as a proportion of the same bone in the control skeleton. The results from different bones when plotted together show the size distribution of the cattle in the archaeological sample. The top plot shows two peaks among the 7th-millennium cattle, which are interpreted as female and male wild cattle. The lower plot, of 6th-millennium cattle, shows a decrease in size, typical of domestication, and a high proportion of females, showing a much greater selectivity than in the earlier deposits.

47

Evidence for husbandry practices

We must presume that the stimulus for domestication was a desire to control food resources and reduce the seasonal stress on human groups. The dramatic increase in population and the development of civilisations since would seem to indicate that it was a very successful strategy for food production. But, whereas in the past hunters had exploited their prey for hides, meat, fat, sinews and bone, pastoralism is generally geared to the serious exploitation of the living animal as a food resource. Milk, butter, cheese, yoghurt, blood and wool (known as secondary products) are all renewable resources that do not require the slaughter of the animal. A new set of questions is therefore asked of the bone assemblages.

As in earlier periods, evaluating the importance of any individual species is one of the primary objectives of the analysis. This may be in order to determine which of the domestic species was most important to the community, but it may also be to measure the contribution made by the non-domestic species. Typically this information can be extracted by a number of methods. The four common alternatives are to count the identified bones of each species; to weigh them; to calculate the smallest number of each species (minimum number of individuals, or MNI) that could possibly be represented by the bones in the sample; and to count the number of layers from the same archaeological period which contain the same species. The results will be different for each method (fig. **32**). When comparing the evidence from two different excavations it is important to use only the results achieved by similar methods. The MNI figures essentially represent the relative number of each species killed; the weight represents dietary or meat contribution –since there is a relationship between bone weight and carcass weight; the fragment method falls between and probably most closely represents the number of 'joints' or units of meat of each species. The figures can then be used to calculate the food contribution of each species, which is done by multiplying by an index that relates to the meat weight of each species. However, given the taphonomic problems for many samples, it is wise not to treat these results too precisely.

The relative importance of the domestic species varies even between contemporary sites and often changes through time on any one site. These changes can

Species	Fragment nos (%)	Weight (%)	MNI$_1$ (%)	MNI$_2$ (%)
Horse	0.1	0.54	0.6	1.2
Cattle	49.6	71.8	26.4	23.4
Sheep or goat	30.3	15.6	33.2	26.6
Pig	14.4	11.6	24.1	21.4
Dog	0.06	0.02	0.5	0.5
Cat	0.3	0.01	1.6	1.4
Red deer	0.03	0.04	0.6	0.7
Roe deer	0.02	0.01	0.3	0.4
Goose	0.74	0.16	2.0	5.7
Chicken	1.65	0.17	7.9	11.0
Wild birds	0.1	0.01	2.8	1.8
Fish	2.7	0.04	?	5.9

32 The bones from middle Saxon deposits in Southampton, England, were quantified in four different ways: the number of fragments of each species; the total weight of the bones of each species; the minimum number of individuals (MNI) represented among all the bones of each species (MNI$_1$); and the cumulative total of the MNI for each species in each feature (MNI$_2$).

be readily illustrated using any of the quantification methods described above.

There is an important contrast in a bone assemblage of domestic animals between the exploitation of a live herd for secondary products and that of the animal itself. The difference results in very specific patterns of husbandry which it is believed can be identified among the bone remains. Husbandry for meat production might involve a herd or flock from which excess young males are removed to a market, at their optimum size, with only a limited number being left to breed. Some young females may also be culled, but many will be kept to breed and will only be slaughtered when they cease to be productive. Therefore, a bone assemblage with a high proportion of animals of one or two years of age and a number of old adults might be interpreted as reflecting the consumer or market end of a husbandry geared to meat production, particularly if it could be shown that in the main the young animals were males and the adults females.

A dairy herd produces a different pattern. Very young animals, mainly males, may be killed once lactation has been established in the female. The herd or flock is therefore made up of adult females producing milk, which are only slaughtered when they fail to reproduce, and a small number of breeding males. This model would predict relatively high numbers of bones indicating animals below six months, and an adult sample dominated by females. It should be noted that in the past cattle, sheep and goats produced milk for a shorter period and in much smaller quantities than do modern animals. Lactation in cattle probably lasted little more than six months and the presence of the calf would normally have been needed to initiate and maintain lactation. There is considerable argument over whether this is an appropriate model, many believing that the milk was shared between young and humans, and that there was no necessity to kill the offspring, which could have been reared and fattened for slaughter at a more productive age. It is worth noting that a high proportion of animals that died within their first six months can also be interpreted as an autumn cull – the removal of unwanted young stock from a small flock or herd before the winter, on account of limitations in the available winter fodder or stalls to accommodate them.

The production of wool, as the primary resource of a flock of sheep or goats, has yet another model. The fleece is normally taken off animals between two and six years of age. It is at its finest when the animal is young and becomes progressively more hairy, rather than woolly, as the animals age. In a sheep flock the young males are castrated to prevent their normal aggressive seasonal behaviour, only a few rams being left intact, and both sexes are kept until their wool quality drops. The slaughter pattern from a wool flock is therefore expected to be almost entirely of adults, including both females and castrated males.

In many communities such specialised husbandry practices are of relatively recent origin, and were developed to supply large markets such as towns. We can expect many human groups to practise a mixed pattern of husbandry, which varies in response to the seasonal needs for a food supply for both the humans and the animals. It is also important to understand that the pattern reflected by the bones on a farm, with a herd of cattle being kept for meat to supply the market, will be different to that of the town thus supplied. The latter will have the product of the 'industry', while the farm is more likely to butcher its old or injured unmarketable stock, and may well also include the bones of young animals that were stillborn or died shortly after birth.

Cultural patterns, rather than subsistence needs, might also be significant. Where, for example, cattle are a major status symbol, as among the Masai of

Kenya today, very few young animals are killed, because the maintenance of the herd size is so important. The killing of an animal is thus either a measure of desperation or an indication of great status or feasting.

At the Bronze Age site of Grimes Graves, England, 46 per cent of the cattle jaws indicated animals under six months, and 27 per cent animals over three years. An interpretation of a ratio of 6:1 females to males among the twenty-nine measured adult metacarpals shows that the assemblage conforms to the model proposed for a dairy herd. An example of the controversies that exist in the interpretation of bones is shown by the comparison of this conclusion with that of a researcher studying Irish Iron Age and early Christian material. One Iron Age site, in which approximately 53 per cent of the cattle were killed before six months, and a further 18 per cent at six months, follows the same pattern, i.e. the dairy model. However, documentary evidence for the early Christian period in Ireland strongly indicates that dairying was of major importance and suggests that the absence of the calf stopped the cow letting down her milk, and therefore if calves were killed at very young ages it could not be a dairy herd. This would indicate a different model for dairying, in which the evidence from such a herd would show very few animals of less than six months. The Irish early Christian sites produced evidence to show that less than 13 per cent of the cattle were slaughtered before six months, with the majority of animals killed between seven and thirty-six months, thus fitting the documentary model. Since a young age profile has been used to suggest dairying on sites of the early Neolithic period in central Europe, the reconsideration of these models is important.

At an early medieval site at Birsay, Orkney, the sheep bones, which are of a species used for milk production in many parts of the world, show this same pattern of high mortality among the young animals. Here this has been seen as evidence of high infant mortality as a result of the reduction of stock numbers before winter, probably necessitated by limited winter fodder. However, this interpretation, known as 'autumn killing' and once fashionable, is not currently in vogue. Interpretation is thus rarely clear cut, and many other lines of evidence – documentary, geographical, climatic or archaeological – may have to be used in order to develop the interpretation of the bone data.

The interpretation of the importance of an individual species often demands information other than just the species abundance. Urban centres in Britain during the late Saxon and medieval periods show an increasing dominance of sheep bones. There is a change in the bone assemblages from a predominance of cattle (80–90 per cent of fragments) to medieval samples where sheep make up 60 per cent or more of the bones. While showing a clear change in the importance of these two species to the diet of town-dwellers in England, the underlying reason for this change is only clear when the age structure of the sheep is analysed. The application of the techniques already described shows that the majority of the sheep bones derive from adults (animals of three years and over), an age structure consistent with the model for wool production. In fact, this change reflects the major expansion of the English wool trade during the medieval period and its consequent impact on meat supplies. A tendency is seen in the post-medieval period for the proportions of sheep to drop as beef cattle reassert their contribution to the English diet.

Sometimes changes in the species proportions may reflect environmental changes or differences in the potential of geographic areas. Norse sites in Greenland have a high proportion of goat bones, much higher than equivalent sites in

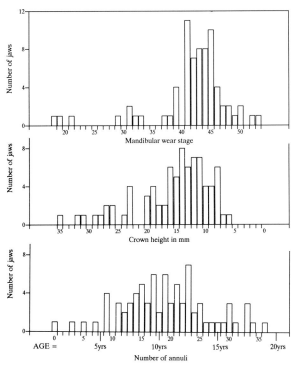

33 Various methods are available for estimating the age of animals from their teeth: the pattern of wear on the occluding (grinding) surface can be recorded (mandibular wear stage); the height of the crown of the tooth can be measured; or the teeth can be sectioned and the 'annual' lines counted. These methods were compared on a sample of 75 Roman cattle jaws from Castle Street, Carlisle, England. The 'annuli' are presumed to be the most accurate and show a very marked adult distribution, with few animals under 5 years and some individuals over 15 years old.

Iceland, from where the settlers probably came. This is seen as a response to the copse-herb vegetation of Greenland, which goats can digest but sheep cannot, i.e. an environmentally controlled choice rather than a cultural one.

As well as recognising and interpreting the significance through time of changes in species abundance, we can also observe these changes within a species. On many Roman fort and urban sites in Britain, the cattle jaws show an age structure indicating very few animals killed before two years old and a great many old animals (see fig. **33**). This pattern is seen in Roman London and contrasts with evidence from the Middle Saxon town where 50 per cent of the animals had been killed by two years of age. Both sites are urban, both represent the waste from domestic consumption, but the Saxon example suggests beef production, while the Roman one is more typical of a dairy herd or draught animals. Unfortunately the jaws cannot be sexed, so we are unable to discover how many females or males are present. Although the market is similar, the economic demands must have been different. Perhaps a much higher proportion of Roman cattle were kept for milking and as plough oxen, since cereal cultivation for grain export was an important element in the Roman economy.

Fishing, trade and distribution

There are significant differences in the proportion of wild as against domestic resources on many sites. In Iron Age farming communities in Britain the consumption of wild game was seemingly very small, often less than 1 per cent of all the bones recovered. However, on coastal sites the opportunity to exploit resources such as sea birds, their eggs and fish introduces a much greater variety to

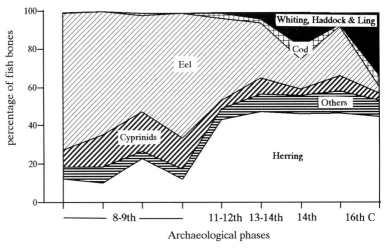

34 The abundance of freshwater fish and eels diminishes sharply after the Saxon period at Fishergate, York, and from the 11th century onwards the proportion of marine species – particularly herring and members of the cod family – rises. These changes are probably a reflection of the developing commercial fisheries, the demand for fish in major towns, and the adherence to fish on certain religious days.

the bone assemblages. In some areas these resources may have been a very important element of the diet and economy.

Although humans have been fishing for thousands of years, the species exploited have changed as fishing and boat technology and the needs of the market have developed. One of the major changes that took place in medieval Europe was the development of the white and stockfish industry. Evidence for the development of trade in marine fish can be found in many urban settlements (fig. **34**). It is thought that the whitefish were gutted, de-headed, sometimes filleted, then dried or salted and exported to population centres. The absence of head bones but not the vertebrae is seen as evidence of this trade, the processing having taken place elsewhere; but it may also illustrate that the fishmongers gutted and filleted the fish before sale. On an early medieval site at Freswick, on the north-east coast of Scotland, an enormous midden stretching for over 100 metres along the dunes contained mainly bones of the cod family. Over 90 per cent by weight of the bone from the soil samples was fish. Such a superabundance suggests that not only did this community eat fish, but that it might well have been a fishing village that caught, gutted, filleted, smoked or salted fish for export to markets in the south or even on the Continent.

There is other evidence for the distribution of food besides that relating to the obvious need to supply the developing towns. The presence on some sites of age-selected culls suggests a level of control over the food supply unlikely at a commercial market stall. The age structure of the pig bones (fig. **35**) from early medieval levels at Westminster Abbey, London, shows a marked preference for individuals killed between twelve and twenty-four months, as well as 'sucking pigs' (animals not yet weaned). This could only have resulted from controlled selection from the abbey herds for supply to the abbey, and shows consumption of the choicest meat – a high level of selectivity only possible while the animals were unbutchered or alive. Long-distance transport of food resources on the hoof is probably much more common than can be proved from the archaeological remains.

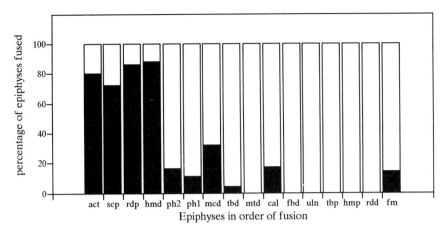

35 The pig epiphyses from Westminster Abbey have been arranged in the approximate order in which they fuse during life, with those that fuse first on the left. Each bar indicates the percentage of one particular epiphysis which had fused. Between 15 and 20 per cent of the pigs had no epiphyses fused and were therefore sucking pigs or neonates that died within a few weeks of birth. About 65 per cent were killed after the fusion of the distal humerus (**hmd**), which has normally fused by about 12 months, but before the next epiphysis, the 2nd phalanx (**ph2**), which fuses by the end of the second year.

Material from a seventeenth-century Dutch whaling station at Smeerenburg, Spitzbergen, has been excavated. The keeping of domestic herbivores is not possible on these islands and all the domestic meat was imported from the Netherlands, where it had been butchered, salted and packed in barrels for shipping. The absence of skulls in the sample reflects the difficulty of transport and low food value of the head, mirroring the decisions of prehistoric hunters at a kill site. Also absent were the bones of the feet, elements of no value to the whaling station. The remainder of the skeleton is present, indicating that individual carcasses were butchered and packed specifically for this station, with no selectivity regarding meat or joint.

Such barrelled food supplies must have been quite common in the past. Finds amongst the cargo of a wrecked Phoenician vessel, for example, included salted pork joints in a barrel. Similar long-distance transport is suggested by finds of exotic animals: examples from archaeological deposits of various dates in London include swordfish, turtle, barbary ape, capuchin and vervet monkeys, although some of these are unlikely to have been eaten, and were probably transported alive to be sold as pets or curiosities.

A representation of skeletal elements similar to those used to suggest either kill sites or camps on prehistoric excavations are used on historic sites to suggest animals bred and killed on the premises or butchered and marketed as food. These models are used to indicate either a producer or a consumer site. Such analyses are important for understanding whether a site is subsisting or generating a surplus for distribution. A model of production, distribution, butchery and redistribution of meat on the joint is proposed for the supply of urban or consumer sites. Low proportions of skulls and feet, along with heavily butchered bones, are seen as evidence of the domestic consumption of meat purchased already jointed. A concentration on cattle, sheep and pigs, with a low diversity and abundance of other species, is also characteristic.

In most medieval and post-medieval levels on many European town sites there is a contrast between the age structure and skeletal representation of pigs and those of sheep and cattle. The pig bones often include bones from animals that died shortly after birth, suggesting pig breeding on the site. The presence of all parts of the carcass, including skulls and feet, is evidence of whole carcasses being butchered. This is interpreted as evidence of 'backyard' farming and is frequently found in association with the bones of chickens, ducks and geese, and occasional finds of whole uneaten eggs. There are various medieval ordinances aimed at preventing pigs from feeding on the rubbish lying around towns, and untended pigs could be given to hospitals for food. Cattle show a pattern more consistent with the purchase of butchered joints, with no very young animals. It was the absence of this backyard farming pattern and the low diversity of species at eighth/ninth-century York that led to the suggestion that the settlement at Fishergate was a trading post, supplied with all its food needs by a central authority. In contrast its successor, the tenth/eleventh-century settlement at Coppergate, produced evidence of animal keeping, as do contemporary deposits in Southampton and London.

Wealth, status and culture

If we can recognise differences at this level of detail, can we also recognise evidence for status or wealth? There are numerous examples supporting this sort

	Westminster Abbey (11th C)	Barnard Castle (15th C)		Westminster Abbey (11th C)	Barnard Castle (15th C)
Cattle	769	24	Roker	334	
Sheep	535	36	Ray family	238	7
Pig	615	32	Sturgeon	21	
Red deer	4	2	Eel	571	99
Roe deer	18	2	Herring	2923	425
Fallow deer		9	Salmon	1	
Hare	7	7	Trout/Salmon	80	45
Rabbit	2	1	Smelt	1614	
Dolphin	1		Pike	198	8
Chicken	205	26	Trench	5	
Domestic goose	12	8	Bream	5	
Wild goose sp.	4		Barbel	4	
Domestic duck	17		Dace	27	
Teal	2		Chub	1	
Widgeon	1		Dace/Chub	74	
Pintail	1	1	Roach	64	
Tufted duck	3		Cyprinidae	646	1
Goldeneye	1		Cod	57	33
Moorhen		4	Haddock	19	17
Rock/Stock dove	5	4	Whiting	806	1
Fieldfare	1	9	Ling	1	6
Blackbird	4		Cod family	54	8
Song thrush/Redwing	3	2	Conger eel		9
Woodcock	8		Tub gurnard	20	
Snipe	1		Gurnard family	87	7
Redshank		1	Bass		4
Red grouse		1	Mackerel		45
Partridge		4	Brill/Turbot	9	4
White stork	1		Plaice	221	
Common crane	1		Flounder	53	
			Plaice/Flounder	1221	12

36 These two medieval assemblages show a very wide diversity of probable food species. This diversity and the occurrence of species such as deer and sturgeon indicate high status. Many of these species were only identified from samples which were sieved.

of conclusion. For instance, deer remains are found more often on medieval castle and palace sites in England than in the towns and villages, illustrating that hunting deer was prohibited to the majority of the population at this time. In medieval deposits excavated within the castle at Barnard Castle, over 20 per cent of the identified bones were deer.

Diversity is a major criterion, particularly if many species had to be brought from some distance. The contents of the fifteenth-century kitchen drains at Barnard Castle and the rubbish from the eleventh-century levels at Westminster Abbey (fig. **36**) both illustrate this. The wide variety of food on the tables of the aristocracy, especially marine fish transported 60 km or more, would be difficult to match in our most expensive modern restaurants.

Excavations at Great Zimbabwe, dating from between AD 1150 and 1550, have uncovered separate areas believed to be for commoners, the élite and royalty. Almost all of the bones found are of cattle, but the age structure of those in the commoners' area shows that only about 33 per cent were slaughtered when under thirty months, with the remainder adult. In the midden beneath the Acropolis, and in another midden associated with royal quarters, over 75 per cent of the cattle were killed by thirty months. This shows a preferential selection of prime cattle associated with high-status areas; such a cull may have been used by the kings to show off their status. The importance of cattle to these communities in terms of status is further indicated by the fifteenth- and sixteenth-century settlement at Manekweni, another site in Zimbabwe; there, as one moves away from the central royal enclosure to the periphery, the abundance of cattle relative to sheep and goats decreases in the middens.

A dramatic example of the level of social detail that can be obtained from bone analyses is given by the study of a hundred cesspits from excavations of seventeenth- and eighteenth-century tenements at Waterlooplein, Amsterdam. The analyses show the absence or near absence of pork bones, an absence of the hind limb bones of cattle, a lack of calves, and high numbers of chicken bones. Such an assemblage can be described as kosher and indicates the presence of Jewish households. This was confirmed by the presence of many lead seals, some attached to chicken leg bones: these were stamped with the day of the week the chicken were butchered and show that the meat is kosher. It was possible to establish where these households were concentrated and which were the wealthiest, identified by the high percentages of tuna, herring, garfish, pike, perch and salmon in the cesspits. Even changes in the status of individual households could be identified, by comparing cesspits of different dates within the same tenement.

— 6 —

Industries, Crafts and Ritual Deposits

Animal bones can often give us evidence of activities incidental or secondary to food and diet. Such activities may relate to industries that process animal carcasses, to manufacturing crafts, or even to religious ceremonies.

Slaughter yards and craft workshops

The slaughter and butchery of a carcass generates many secondary products, and the identification of slaughterhouses or butchers is often a simple exercise. In the days before refrigeration domestic animals were always walked to market and slaughtered, cattle sometimes being driven many miles to the best markets. In a developed urban society, slaughtering and the initial butchery would be done in the same place to enable the removal of secondary products that could be sold on elsewhere. The most obvious of these products are the horns, hide and bones. Evidence of this primary butchering is characterised by large numbers of skulls, often split to extract the brain. In medieval and post-medieval London, a number of sites with the remains of cattle skulls occur south of the river in Southwark. The siting of slaughterhouses here probably indicates an embargo on driving cattle across London Bridge in order to prevent the accumulation of foul-smelling offal and blood in the City. Similar examples elsewhere include debris in the ditch of the Roman fortress at Exeter, where most of the skulls were missing their horn-cores (the bones which the horn itself sheaths), indicating the intention of using the horn before disposal.

Collections of horn-cores are common in European towns, sometimes occurring in dumps of hundreds or even thousands. The cores, the waste from the horn industry, were sometimes sold or passed on and used to build walls or to line pits and drains in late medieval and post-medieval times. Many of these cores show the marks of the chop which removed them from the skull. This blow was normally struck from the back or below the horn, rather than on the top of the skull. Little evidence exists for the activity of actually working the horn, or for the items produced, such as spoons, vessels or lanterns, since horn normally degrades in the soil. Sometimes the horn was worked while still attached to the horn-core. This produced sawn segments of the horn-core, and these and other waste are found from the Roman period onwards – providing evidence of horners in many European towns.

Horners may have worked alongside the skinners and tanners, although the latter were banned from many town centres in the medieval period because of the smell generated by their work. In the past it appears that when the hides were skinned from the carcass the feet were left attached and the limbs dismembered at the knuckle or ankle. Collections of bones that show a predominance of these foot bones can be interpreted as waste from tanning if unassociated with other primary butchery waste. The juxtaposition of a series of eighteenth-century tanning pits at Walmgate, York, with hundreds of metapodials and phalanges of sheep is by association convincing evidence that this type of bone assemblage is waste from tanning. Similar associations have been found at other sites and individual examples are not uncommon in the literature, although they are not always interpreted as evidence of tanning. An early medieval site at Aldwark, York, produced an abundance of goat skulls, jaws and feet bones. The age profile obtained from the teeth showed a careful selection of animals of about two and a half years old which were almost exclusively male, a factor evident from the horn-core measurements. In this example it seems likely that the bones represent waste from both a horner's workshop and either a skinner preparing the goat-skins or a tanner preparing the hides.

The identification of the preparation of skins rather than leather is not possible from the bone debris, since both crafts will generate the same waste. The same is not true for similar trades dealing with fur-bearing or exotic animals. A post-medieval deposit in central London produced skull and jaw fragments of bears, foxes and leopards. Some of these were chopped in a manner that suggests they derive from a skin to which the skull was still attached, presumably as display pieces. Archaeological finds of the foot bones of bears are normally interpreted as deriving from skins, and the ocurrence of these bones in a number of Iron Age graves suggests the burial of the body wrapped in, covered by or laid on a bearskin.

Evidence for trade in furs is a little easier to interpret. Foot bones are often left in the skins until the fur is worked. A furrier might therefore be expected to generate as waste the bones of the feet of the skins being used. These bones may well bear the traces of fine cuts associated with skinning them out with as little damage to the skin as possible. A very early archaeological example is afforded by the numerous pine marten bones found on the Mesolithic site at Tybrind Vig, Denmark. The skulls showed skinning cuts, but there were no signs of butchery to suggest that the animals were also eaten. Other examples are rare, but occasional finds of pine martens in Roman and medieval towns most probably indicate pelts. A small group of pine marten foot bones from eighth/ninth century levels at Fishergate, York, including one bone bearing knife cuts, was seen as evidence of pelts, and a similar conclusion was reached for squirrel foot bones from two other York sites of ninth/tenth- and fourteenth-century date.

Another commercial use of the waste from the butchering process is indicated by a number of similar collections found on Roman sites from Carlisle in England to Augst in Switzerland. These collections are dominated by the long bones and ankle bones of cattle limbs, almost to the exclusion of other bones. Most of these bones are very heavily butchered and fragmented. In the sample from Carlisle an estimated total of nearly 1500 animals was represented by this waste: the quantity and character of the bone assemblages clearly indicate large-scale processing.

When originally reported from the Roman castellum at Zwammerdam, Holland, they were interpreted as the waste from a soup kitchen, and at Augst as a glue factory. There is little to justify the exclusion of other bones from a soup kitchen and it seems more probable that the bones were boiled to extract the bone grease, oils and marrow fats that are concentrated in the marrow cavities of the long bones and the ankle joints.

Bone and antler working

The use of bone as a raw material for the manufacture of tools and other objects is likely to have as long a history as the use of stone tools. Many of the weapons which prehistoric people used for hunting game were made from the bones of the animals they hunted. The character of the bones and teeth available to them varied appreciably in its physical properties. The hardness of ivory and the strength and elasticity of bone and antler were important considerations in the ways they were used. The earliest tools, recognised by the signs of wear and polish, were made from bone splinters resulting from smashing the bones to extract the marrow. By the late Palaeolithic and Mesolithic periods, bone working was more refined and the harpoons, arrowheads and decorative objects required considerable skill (fig. **37**). Antler was grooved lengthwise and then split to remove long pieces of the hard outer layer, which could then be worked to make points or other implements. Ivory spears found in late Palaeolithic Russian burials were made from the ivory of mammoths, whose tusks were strongly curved, so that a method must have been developed by these people to straighten them. Ivory was often used for decorative objects. One of the earliest

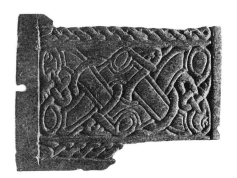
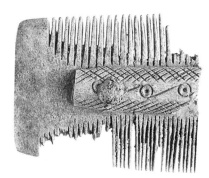
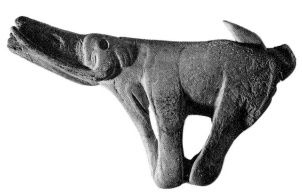

37 Many bone artefacts illustrate the ritual, decorative and functional use of bone. These three examples include a medieval decorative bone plate, a Norse comb and a Palaeolithic spear-thrower.

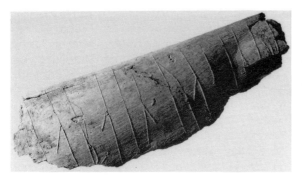

38 Many bone fragments are inscribed with graffiti or used as trial pieces for designs and decorations. This cow rib from Norse excavations at Earls Bu, Orkney, carries a rune which reads '...bone was in ...'. We are unfortunately none the wiser.

representations of the human form, seen as an earth mother fertility figure, was made from mammoth ivory. Some early drawings and inscriptions are scratched on pieces of bone (fig. **38**).

Bone objects or tools are common finds on many excavations of the prehistoric period, but identifiable workshops only become recognisable in the Roman and early medieval periods. Sawn offcuts and waste pieces become much more common and, although some objects were almost certainly made when needed from pieces of waste food bone, a professional class of craftsmen can be deduced from both the quality of objects being manufactured (fig. **37**) and the waste from their workshops (fig. **39**). Antler waste from comb workshops comprises offcuts of the crown and burr, flakes or shavings, some tines, broken or poorly cut pieces originally intended for use, and trial pieces (bone pieces carved with designs as a 'roughout'). Examples of such workshops have been found in York, Southampton, Hedeby, Ribe, Staré Mesto, Staraja Ladoga and other early European towns.

Not all bones are useful, but plate-like bones such as the shoulder blade (scapula), jaw and ribs were frequently used for flat objects, playing pieces or decorative bone plaques. The shafts of long bones, particularly the metapodial

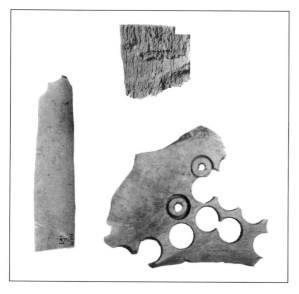

39 Bone-working waste, including offcuts from bones used in comb-making, antler shavings and bead making.

(cannon) bones of animals such as cattle, horses and deer, are used for manufacturing pins, awls and needles, the waste being the sawn ends of the bones. Such groups of waste are not uncommon in early medieval towns. The rarest materials, and therefore the most valuable, such as ivory, are often used for purely decorative items. Although objects of elephant and walrus ivory are found throughout this period, evidence for ivory workshops before the post-medieval period has not been found. A collection of ivory waste from a workshop manufacturing combs and knife-handles has been found near the Tower of London. The presence of waste pieces on other sites nearby suggests that this area might have had a number of workshops handling ivory.

Religion and ritual deposits

Animals are of major importance to all societies and many cultures deify them or associate rituals or religious significance with them. Although relatively rare, there are examples of bone samples which can be interpreted in terms of ritual or religious behaviour. Human burials involving animals have been found. At Mehrgarh in Baluchistan, a human burial of the eighth millennium BC included five goat kids; and at Ein Mallah in northern Israel, at an even earlier date, a puppy of either wolf or dog was found placed below the left hand of a buried body. The veneration of animals within religious cults is illustrated by the bird and cat mummies from Egyptian tombs. At Çatal Hüyük, a sixth-millennium BC shrine had rows of the horn-cores of aurochsen set in clay in a bench. Most of the carcass of a Bronze Age aurochs was found in a pit near Heathrow, west London (fig. **40**). The carcass had been partially dismembered and the bones laid in a pile in the pit. Six barbed and tanged arrowheads were found among the bones and the skull was laid on the top of the rest of the carcass. Only a few bones appear to be missing and the assemblage seems to be a ritual deposit rather than just the contents of a pit trap.

Animal sacrifices are also present in the archaeological record. The deliberate killing of domestic species and their burial is suggested by the very high incidence of unusual animal deposits, such as articulated skeletons, in the 891 pits excavated at the Iron Age hillfort at Danebury, Hampshire. Nearly 18 per cent of these pits contained such deposits, and several of the skeletons are associated with stones or sling stones, or lie at the bottom of the pit as if deliberately placed there. These burials include horses, dogs, cattle, sheep, pigs and a goat. The sheer number of these deposits lends them significance, and it is possible that many relate to sacrifical practices at the hillfort. Rather clearer examples of sacrifice are found at temple or tomb excavations. The bone remains from the Iron Age and Roman temple at Uley, Gloucestershire, largely comprised two species, the goat and the chicken. Classical sources indicate that the species and time of sacrifice varied with the deity.

Excavations of tombs at Kerma in Sudan dating from the second and third millennium BC revealed many sheep, goat and occasionally dog sacrifices. Some 50 per cent of the bones from the town site are cattle, but no cattle sacrifices are found in the tombs, although frontal bones and attached horn-cores (known as bucrania) were laid out on the south side looking towards the graves. At one tomb these bucrania were arranged with the bulls to the front and cows, some with calves, behind. The age range of the cattle and this arrangement around the tomb suggested the simultaneous killing of a herd as a sacrifice at the time of

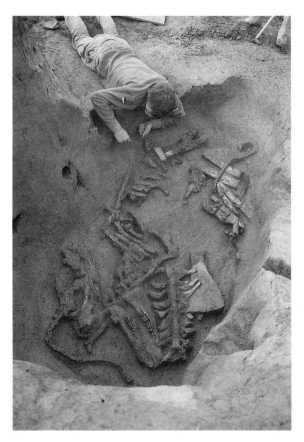

40 This Bronze Age aurochs lies in a pit at Holloway Lane, west London. The soil conditions were acidic and the skull (which was laid on top) has completely disappeared, leaving only the teeth *in situ*. The carcass is incomplete, was partially dismembered, and has six barbed and tanged arrowheads associated with it. It shows the effect of the burial environment on the survival of bone, and is an example of a ritual deposit.

burial. This would have been extremely costly to the community and an alternative explanation suggests that the 'herd' was composed of live cattle, sent from many places around Kerma and beyond as a tribute and then sacrificed. The probability that the burial was accompanied by feasting is suggested by the absence of cattle bucrania from the town sample, the animals being eaten in the town after the sacrifice and placement of the bucrania at the tomb.

There are many other examples of ritual or superstitious rites associated with animals. Skulls are still buried under floors or foundations, and cats and rats were often walled up in houses in the seventeenth and eighteenth centuries. However, because we are so far removed from the people who made these deposits, it is often difficult for us to understand their significance.

Postscript

The importance of animal bones to the archaeologist is often underestimated, even within the profession. Life itself is only sustained through eating, and, whether prehistoric human, or medieval merchant, food – its procurement, cultivation or supply – is essential. Animal products are a major element of this food and in early periods the majority of the population was involved in food production for much of the time. The animal bones found on occupation sites therefore reflect, at various levels, a great deal about the life of past peoples, and those who are interested in the past ignore this at their peril.

I have tried to illustrate how seemingly uninspiring fragments of bone can yield information on a wide range of topics of interest to archaeologists: the age of a site, the prevailing climate, the character of the surrounding environment, hunting methods and prey selection, season of occupation, early domestication, human diet, animal husbandry practices, trade, economics, social status, religion and ritual (among others). These are the end products of a methodical and precise analysis of all the fragments of animal bone collected from an excavation, any one of which 'might' indicate the species from which it derived, the age, sex, size and approximate weight of the animal itself, and perhaps even whether it had been injured in life, how it was killed, and whether it was a working, domestic or wild animal. To make such conclusions requires the consideration of many problems, some soluble and others more difficult to assess. Foremost amongst these are the recovery methods of the excavators, which can introduce a bias, particularly against small bones, if care and methodical sampling procedures are not used, and the taphonomic processes that acted upon the bones after deposition, many of which can lead to the total destruction of the bones.

New techniques and analytical methods can be expected to extend even further the contribution that animal bones can make to interpreting the past. The subject has already become so wide that researchers within the discipline have become specialists in geographic regions or time periods. Despite the variety of areas in which animal bones can contribute to the archaeological interpretation of the past, one of their most important features is that they often illuminate aspects of everyday life rather than the more dramatic religious and cultural information derived from other lines of archaeological evidence. We learn about people – their preferences, food and daily life – from animal bones in a way that can sometimes bring the past alive more directly than visiting monuments or exhibitions of museum artefacts. This shows the necessity of tackling all possible lines of archaeological enquiry if a clear and complete picture of life in the past is to be painted. It is perhaps the multifarious evidence to be gained from the physical sciences, natural sciences, social sciences, economics, history and art combined which makes archaeology and interpreting the past so exciting.

Further Reading

Baker, J. and Brothwell, D. *Animal Diseases in Archaeology*. Academic Press, London, 1980.
Barton, N., Roberts, A.J. and Roe, D.A. (eds). *The Late Glacial in north-west Europe*, CBA Res. Rep. 77, 1991.
Binford, L.R. *Bones, Ancient Men and Modern Myths*. Academic Press, London, 1981.
Brain, C.K. *The Hunters or the Hunted?* University of Chicago Press, Chicago, 1981.
Clutton-Brock, J. and Grigson, C. (eds). *Animals and Archaeology* 1, BAR Int. Ser. 163, Oxford, 1983.
Cohen, A. and Serjeantson, D. *A Manual for the Identification of Bird's Bones from Archaeological Sites*. Alan Cohen, London, 1986.
Davis, S.J.M. *The Archaeology of Animals*. Batsford, London, 1987.
Driesch, A. von den. *A Guide to the Measurement of Animal Bones from Archaeological Sites*. Peabody Museum, Cambridge, Mass., 1976.
Grayson, D.K. *Quantitative Zooarchaeology*. Academic Press, New York, 1984.
Hesse, B. and Wapnish, P. *Animal Bone Archaeology*. Taraxacum, Washington, DC, 1985.
Hillson, S. *Mammal Bones and Teeth: An Introductory Guide to Methods of Identification*. Institute of Archaeology, University College London Press, 1992.
Klein, R.G. and Cruz-Uribe, K. *The Analysis of Animal Bones from Archaeological Sites*. University of Chicago Press, Chicago, 1984.
MacGregor, A. *Bone, Antler, Ivory and Horn*. Croom Helm, Beckenham, Kent, 1985.
Olsen, S.J. *Osteology for the Archaeologist. No. 3: The American Mastodon and the Woolly Mammoth and No. 4: North American Birds*. Peabody Museum, Cambridge, Mass., 1972.
Schmid, E. *Atlas of Animal Bones for Prehistorians, Archaeologists and Quaternary Geologists*. Elsevier, Amsterdam, 1972.
Shipman, P. *Life History of a Fossil: An Introduction to Taphonomy and Paleoecology*. Harvard University Press, Cambridge, Mass., 1981.
Sutcliffe, A.J. *On the Track of Ice Age Mammals*. Natural History Museum, London, 1985.
Walker, R. *A Guide to Post-cranial Bones of East African Animals*. Hylochoerus Press, Norwich, Norfolk, 1985.
Wheeler, A. and Jones, A.K.G. *Fishes*. Cambridge University Press, Cambridge, 1989.

Additional references related to the text and figures

Unpublished reports on London sites can be found in the archive of the Environmental Archaeology Section, Museum of London.

CHAPTER 1
Rackham, D.J., *Mid-Devensian Mammals in Britain*. Unpublished M.Sc. Thesis, University of Birmingham (Isleworth), 1982.
Rackham, D.J., in B. Wilson, C. Grigson and S. Payne (eds), *Ageing and Sexing Animal Bones from Archaeological Sites*, 73–80 (feral goat bone fusion), 1982.
Rackham, D.J. in E. Cruwys and R.A. Foley (eds), *Teeth and Anthropology*, 149–168 (cementum lines in cattle teeth), 1986.

CHAPTER 2
Clark, J.G.D., *Excavations at Star Carr*, 1954.

CHAPTER 3
Andrews, P., in *Animals and Archaeology* 1, 77–86 (Olduvai Gorge), 1983.
Armitage, P. and West, B. *Trans. London & Middlesex Arch. Soc., 36*, 107–137 (Greyfriars, London), 1985.
Klein, R.G. *Archaeology 28*, 238–47 (Nelson Bay Cave), 1975.

Klein, R.G., in H.J. Deacon, Q.B. Hendey and J.J.N. Lambrechts (eds), *Fynbos palaeoecology: a preliminary synthesis,*, 116–138 (Boomplaas Cave), 1983.
Rackham, D.J., in A.R. Hall and H.K. Kenward (eds), *Environmental Archaeology in the Urban context*, 86–93 (Birsay; Droitwich; Coppergate; Barnard Castle), 1982.

CHAPTER 4
Binford, L.R., *Nunamuit ethnoarchaeology,*, 1978.
Bokelmann, K., in *The Late Glacial in north-west Europe*, 72–81 (Tunnel Valley; Stellmoor; Meiendorf), 1991.
Geddes, D., Guilaine, J., Coularou, J., Le Gall, O. and Martzluff, M., in C. Bonsall (ed.), *The Mesolithic in Europe*, 561–571 (Pyrenees), 1990.
Klein, R.G., *J. Archaeological Science 16, No. 4*, 363–382 (Klasies River Mouth), 1989.
White, T.E., *American Antiquity 17*, 337–338, 1952.

CHAPTER 5
Barker, G., *Anthropozoologica, 16*, 47–52 (Great Zimbabwe, Manekweni), 1992.
Donaldson, A.M., Jones, A.K.G. and Rackham, D.J., *J. British Archaeological Association, CXXXIII*, 86–96 (Barnard Castle), 1980.
IJzereef, F.G., in D. Serjeantson and T. Waldron (eds), *Diet and crafts in Towns*, 41–54 (Waterlooplein, Amsterdam), 1989.
Jones, R.T., Sly, J., Simpson, D., Rackham, J. and Locker, A., *The terrestrial vertebrate remains from the excavations at the castle; Barnard Castle*, Ancient Monuments Report, English Heritage, 1985.
Legge, A.J., in A. Milles, D. Williams and N. Gardner (eds), *The Beginnings of Agriculture*, 217–242 (Grimes Graves), 1989.
McCormick, F., *Emania 8*, 57–59 (Iron Age and Early Christian Ireland), 1991.
McGovern, T.H., in Morris, C.D. and Rackham, D.J. (eds), *Norse and later Settlement and Subsistence in the North Atlantic*, 193–230 (Greenland), 1992.
Morris, C.D. and Rackham, D.J., in *Norse and later Settlement and Subsistence in the North Atlantic*, 43–102 (Freswick), 1992.
O'Connor, T.P., in D.J. Rackham (ed.), *Environment and economy in Anglo-Saxon England* (Fishergate, Coppergate), 1993.
Pipe, A.R., *Anthropozoologica, 16*, 189–190 (London exotics), 1992.
Rackham, D.J., unpublished report (Birsay; Westminster Abbey).
Wijngaarden-Bakker, L.H. van and Pals, J.P., *Early European Exploitation of the Northern Atlantic 800–1700*, 133–151 (Smeerenburg, Spitzbergen), 1981.

CHAPTER 6
Chaix, L. and Grant, A., *Anthropozoologica, 16*, 61–66 (Kerma), 1992.
Clutton-Brock, J., *Domesticated animals from early times* (Çatal Hüyük), 1981.
Grant, A., in B. Cunliffe *Danebury, an Iron Age hillfort in Hampshire*, vol. 2, 496–548 (Danebury), 1984.
Maltby, M., *The animal bones from Exeter 1971–1975* (Exeter), 1979.
O'Connor, T.P., *The Archaeology of York*, 15/1, 1–60 (Walmgate), 1984.
O'Connor, T.P., *The Archaeology of York*, 15/3, 137–207 (Coppergate), 1989.
Pipe, A.R., unpublished report (Southwark).
Rackham, D.J., unpublished report (Aldwark; Castle Street, Carlisle).
Trolle-Lassen, T., *Archaeozoologia, 1(2)*, 85–102 (Tybrind Vig), 1987.
van Mensch, P.J., *Berichten van de Rijksdienst voor het Oudheidkundig Bodemonderzoek 24*, 159–165 (Zwammerdam), 1974.

Index

Figure numbers in bold refer to illustrations